THE
HONEY
PHENOMENON

How This Liquid Gold
HEALS Your Ailing Body

Dr. Joshua Levitt

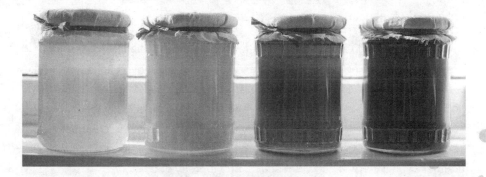

The Healing Powers of Honey

My mother-in-law winced in pain as she cautiously took the bandage off her leg. Three weeks before, she had a large, deep skin cancer removed. The surgical wound had been repeatedly infected and was not healing well at all. Her surgeon had recommended all sorts of different ointments and topical treatments, but nothing was working. Her next step was an appointment with a wound care specialty clinic.

What I saw underneath that bandage was a deep, raw, open wound... it looked like somebody had taken a tablespoon and scooped out a large chunk of her leg. There were a bunch of non-squeamish family members gathered around and everybody, including my mother in law, was shocked at what I said next. I told her that I wanted her to pack the wound with honey.

You've got to understand that this was like the ultimate "practice what you preach moment" for me. Yes, I told my mother-in-law to pack a deep surgical wound with honey. It was also a major "leap of faith" for her - do I trust my naturopathic

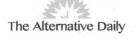

The Alternative Daily

physician son-in-law's advice and fill up a hole in my leg with something I usually only drizzle over oatmeal or spread on toast?!

It should come as no surprise that this story has a happy ending. Mom took my advice and we treated the wound with a topical application of manuka honey. It was apparent within 24 hours that there was progress. We could see granulation tissue developing within the base of the wound, which is evidence that new connective tissue cells and blood vessels are being formed. Then gradually, as you would expect, the healing process continued until the wound healed over completely. All that's left now is a scar… and a pretty good story.

Fact: Honey never, ever goes bad. Archaeologists found 2000-year-old jars of honey in Egyptian tombs and they still tasted amazing!

First Things First

Before we get into the details of all of the science and remarkable research that has been done on the medicinal properties of honey, I welcome you to be in awe of the fact that honey even exists. Here's how it works:

Flowers need help to reproduce. They need to get the pollen from the anthers of one flower to the stigma of another. Bees are perfectly adapted to this task… but they don't do it for free. Flowers that need to be pollinated produce a sweet nectar that lures in the bees with a promise of a sweet treat.

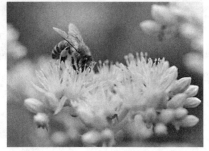

As the bees are gathering this nectar, their bodies get covered in pollen which they carry from one flower to another, pollinating the flowers as they go. The sweet nectar is then brought back to the hive where it is concentrated into this liquid gold… and that's the miracle of honey.

Did you know: Honey bees do a dance when they get back to the hive to tell all the other bees where the flowers are!

A Look Back in Time

Humans have been enamored with honey for thousands of years. In fact, an 8,000-year-old rock drawing found in Spain depicts a honey-seeker robbing a wild hive. Honey has been found buried with Pharaohs in Egypt, and after thousands of years it was still edible.

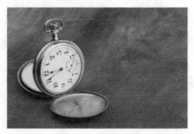

Honey was the most popular ancient Egyptian healing remedy, and was mentioned over 500 times in 900 remedies (Al-Jabri AA. Honey, milk and antibiotics. Afr J Biotechnol.2005;4:1580–1587.)

Ancient Egyptians, Assyrians, Chinese, Romans and Greeks used honey for treating wounds and to heal conditions of the gut. The actual prescription for wound salve dating between 2600 and 2200 BC called for a mixture of grease, honey and lint or fiber. Even ancient physicians recognized the therapeutic value of this natural gift.

Hippocrates himself used honey and vinegar for pain, honey and water for thirst and honey mixed with water and other substances for fever.

Both the Bible and the Qur'an mention the value of honey. The Old Testament refers to the land of Israel as the "land flowing with milk and honey." John the Baptist survived on locusts and honey, and God nourished Jacob with honey from the rock and provided Israel with fine flour, olive oil and honey. The Qur'an mentions that honey is "healing for humankind."

> **Eat honey, my child for it is good.** - Proverbs 24:13

Properties of Honey

Honey contains glucose, fructose, and numerous minerals including calcium, phosphate, sodium chlorine, magnesium and potassium.

According to BeeSource, a typical profile of the sugars in honey looks like this:

- Fructose: 38.2%
- Glucose: 31.3%
- Maltose: 7.1%
- Sucrose: 1.3%
- Water: 17.2%
- Higher sugars: 1.5%
- Ash: 0.2%
- Other/undetermined: 3.2%

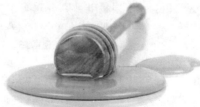

The Alternative Daily

Honey is quite acidic, with a pH between 3.2. and 4.5. This helps prevent the growth of bacteria. It is also loaded with antioxidants. Of course, its exact properties vary depending on the specific flora that was used to produce it, as well as its water content.

Therapeutic properties

Honey is truly a healing gift from nature, and is rich in medicinal properties including:

- **Hygroscopic property:** In its natural state, honey has a very low water content, but it absorbs moisture when exposed to air. This hygroscopic property makes honey highly beneficial to dry skin by allowing it to better retain moisture. It also helps to speed up wound healing time.

- **Antibacterial property:** One especially vital component in honey, glucose oxidase, is an enzyme that produces hydrogen peroxide. Research indicates that this is one of the main reasons why honey seems to have such powerful antibacterial and wound-healing capabilities. The production of hydrogen peroxide is just one of the remarkable ways that honey helps to kill bacteria and heal wounds.

- **Antioxidant property:** Although darker honey generally contains more antioxidant power than light colored, both are still a rich source of valuable antioxidants. Antioxidants go to work against free radicals and encourage new tissue growth. This, in turn, helps expedite healing of damaged tissue and also helps skin appear younger and more radiant.

> *...every spoon of honey contains TINY quantities of these floral flavonoids...usually referred to as antioxidants. There are at least 16 of them found in honey at last count...Trace amounts of these floral flavones exert POWERFUL influences.*

~The Honey Revolution, 2008 p.5

Honey vs. Table Sugar

They're both sweet, right? So don't they have the same effect on my body? This is a common question... many people don't understand that there are significant differences in the way the body responds to honey versus table sugar. Although both honey and sugar contain both glucose and fructose, there are chemical differences in the way that these sugars are linked together.

When table sugar is extracted from sugar cane (or sugar beets) and then processed, the proteins, nitrogen elements, and enzymes found in the natural sugar cane are destroyed.

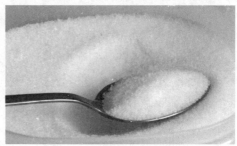

In contrast, honey is a natural sweetener that is only minimally processed, and is loaded with antioxidant and antimicrobial properties.

Table sugar (sucrose) is comprised of two sugar molecules (fructose and glucose) bound together. Before table sugar can be used for energy, we must break it down using an enzyme that will separate these molecules. When bees produce honey, they supply the enzyme needed so we don't have to use our own energy to break the bonds. What a wonderful gift this is!

Table sugar, unlike honey, is void of any vitamins or minerals. This is why it is often referred to as a source of "empty calories." In fact, the calories from table sugar are even worse than empty… they are dangerous. When we consume table sugar in the amounts commonly consumed today, we see clear evidence of increased risks of diabetes and cardiovascular disease.

Gram for gram, honey is sweeter than sugar. This effect allows us to use less honey than table sugar to achieve the same level of sweetness. Although one tablespoon of sugar contains 46 calories and one tablespoon of honey has 64, you can use far less honey than sugar due to its innate and intense sweetness.

Types of Honey

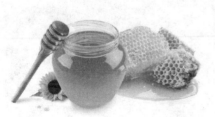

Because bees use the nectar from a variety of plants to make honey, there are many different types of honey, hailing from all over the world. The characteristics, including the aroma, flavor and color of honey, are relative to the specific plant from which it was made.

The following are some popular honey types, as well as blends (mixtures of more than one type of honey):

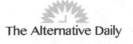

- **Acacia:** Pale in color, almost glass-like, this honey is amongst the most popular of all types and comes from the black locust tree (also called the false "Acacia" tree) native to North America. It has a very mild and sweet flavor which allows it to be used in a variety of ways. Many people enjoy acacia honey in beverages because it does not change the taste of the drink. Although this honey is very sweet, it has a very low sucrose and fructose level, making it a good choice for diabetics.

- **Alfalfa:** Obtained from the purplish flowers of the alfalfa plant, this honey is one of the best substitutes for sugar in tea. It is light in color with a fresh floral scent and is less sweet than some other varieties.

- **Avocado:** If you love fruit, this is the honey for you. Dark in color with a slightly buttery taste, this honey is widely produced in Mexico, Australia and some parts of America. It is often used in dressings and sauces.

- **Blueberry:** Derived from the flowers of blueberry plants, this honey is light amber to amber in color, with the subtle reminder of its origin. Used in sauces and baked goods, this sweet treat is produced mainly in England, as well as in Michigan in the United States

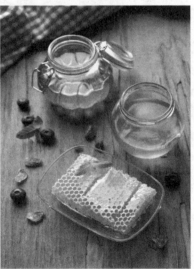

- **Buckwheat:** This honey is the darkest and most strongly-flavored of all honey varieties, and is loaded with iron. Buckwheat honey is particularly popular in Europe. The darker the color, the better the honey.

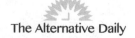

- **Clover:** Although it originated in Canada and New Zealand, clover honey is now available all over the world. This floral-scented honey is generally white to light amber in color and mixes well into salads and baked goods.

- **Fireweed:** The perennial herb that produces the sweet nectar for this honey is grown largely in the Northern and Pacific states, and in Canada. Used mostly for cooking and baking, fireweed honey is also tasty on grilled meat and fish.

- **Manuka:** This popular honey comes from the tea tree bush of New Zealand and has numerous applications. It is the most widely studied honey for medicinal purposes. Manuka honey is prized for its antibacterial properties and, although generally used therapeutically, is completely safe and delicious to eat every day.

- **Orange blossom:** Obtained from orange blossoms, this honey is a light color and has a fruity aroma. With its mild citrus taste, this honey appeals to fruit lovers and pairs well with cheeses.

- **Pumpkin blossom:** Produced from the nectar of a pumpkin blossom, this honey is dark amber in color with a sweet floral fragrance. It is used widely in cooking and is especially nice as a dessert topping.

- **Rainforest:** Rainforest trees found in Australia, Thailand, Tasmania, Brazil and some parts of America provide the nectar for this honey. It is often used in sauces, for baking and is delicious in a warm glass of organic milk.

- **Rata:** This honey is from New Zealand, and is light in color with a sweet, but not strong, taste. Many people use this honey in smoothies and it makes a great addition to energy drinks.

- **Red gum:** This dark honey is loaded with antioxidants and has a strong flavor. It is highly valued for its therapeutic properties, but is also widely enjoyed as a natural sweetener in drinks and food.

- **Rewarewa:** The flowers that produce the nectar for this honey grow in the hills of New Zealand and sport red, needle-like flowers. The honey has a slight caramel taste and leaves a somewhat burnt aftertaste.

- **Pinetree:** This honey also goes by the name of forest honey, tea honey, fir honey and honeydew. It hails from Greece, is loaded with minerals and proteins and has a strong aroma but a delightfully sweet taste. Pinetree honey never crystallizes no matter how long it sits.

- **Sage:** There are a number of different types of sage plant that produce this very light, almost water-white, honey. Due to its very sweet flavor, many people enjoy this honey with cheese.

Did you know: A honey bee visits 50 to 100 flowers during a collection trip.

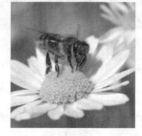

- **Sourwood:** The sourwood tree grows in the Appalachian Mountains, all the way from Southern Pennsylvania to Northern Georgia. With a sweet and spicy aroma and taste, this honey is often used in glazes.

- **Tawari:** This honey is a stunning golden color, and has a sweet butterscotch flavor which allows it to be paired well with gluten-free pancakes and homemade ice cream.

- **Tulip poplar:** The tulip poplar tree has strikingly beautiful blossoms and produces a dark amber honey with a surprisingly mild taste. Many people use this rich honey in cooking and baking.

- **Tupelo:** The trees that produce this sweet honey's nectar have greenish-colored flowers that grow in clusters and eventually turn into berry-like fruit. This honey ranges from white to light amber in color with a slight greenish tint. The flavor is very sweet as this honey is high in fructose.

- **Wildflower:** Because bees collect nectar from a number of different wildflower species, this honey is sometimes called mixed floral or multifloral honey. The taste is fruity with a tangy overtone.

- **Yellow Box:** Native to Australia, and produced from a species of eucalyptus tree, this honey is smooth and used commonly in baking and cooking. It is also a nice addition to a warm cup of tea.

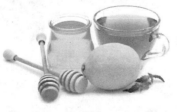

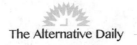

Popular Honey Blends:

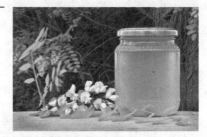

- **Aster:** Light honey produced in the United States that crystallizes quickly.

- **Basswood:** Slightly woody taste and aroma make this honey great for marinades and dressings.

- **Beechwood:** Very dark honey that is often used in sauces and known for its ability to aid in digestion.

- **Blue gum:** With a slightly minty taste, this honey comes from Tasmania and South Australia.

- **Dandelion:** This honey is amber colored and has a very sweet taste. Often used in preparing Chinese medicines and herbal treatments.

- **Eucalyptus:** Different species of eucalyptus make up this honey, which is most often used as a sweetener in tea and coffee.

- **Ironbark:** This amber-colored honey is perfect for baking and adding to smoothies.

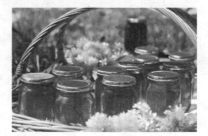

- **Leatherwood:** With a strong, spicy, floral taste, this honey is used in many gourmet products.

- **Linden:** Used extensively in Denmark, this honey is light yellow in color and has a fresh woody aroma. It is well-known for its sedative properties.

- **Macadamia:** Originally found in Australia, this honey is now available in the United States, often in sauces or used to sweeten tea.

- **Neem:** This honey is bitter and not used in baking or cooking, but is valued for its medicinal properties in Ayurvedic medicine as an antibiotic for throat and oral disease, allergies and lowering blood pressure.

> *The careful insect 'midst his works I view, Now from the flowers exhaust the fragrant dew, With golden treasures load his little thighs, And steer his distant journey through the skies.*
>
> ~ John Gay, Rural Sports (canto I, l. 82)

Beware of THIS Honey

Turkish honey, also known as MAD HONEY, or deli bal in Turkey, is made from a rhododendron species that grows in Turkey and can contain a highly poisonous toxin. This dark reddish-colored honey contains a natural neurotoxin that even in small doses can bring on lightheadedness and even hallucinations.

In the early 1700s, this honey was traded with Europeans who mixed it with alcohol for an indistinguishable "buzz." Too much of the honey can cause low blood pressure, numbness, fainting, seizures and even death.

Although there are over 700 species of rhododendron, only a few contain the dangerous grayanotoxin in their nectars. One particular species with the toxin thrives on the slopes around the Black Sea. Because there are few other flowers for bees to collect nectar from, the honey is potent with the toxin.

Turkish honey was even used as an early war tool. In 67 BC, Roman soldiers invaded the Black Sea area under the direction of General Pompey. Those who were still loyal to the reigning King Mithridates placed pieces of mad honeycomb along their path. When the army ate this honey they became intoxicated and were easily slain.

Honey producers in the region claim that the Mad Honey is only a very small amount of the honey that they produce, and that when taken in small doses, it actually has some medicinal value. While the honey is self-regulated in Turkey, it is widely available on the Internet with a whopping price tag of about $166 per pound.

Curious buyer beware: It takes little more than one teaspoon to possibly bring on mad honey poisoning!

> " *The only reason for being a bee that I know of is making honey....and the only reason for making honey is so I can eat it.* "
>
> ~ Winnie the Pooh

One Gift, Many Forms

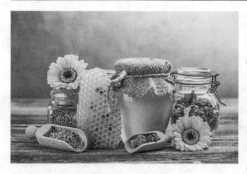

Depending on how honey is processed, it can take on a number of forms, making it suitable for a number of different uses.

Raw honey: Raw honey is honey in its purest state. According to the National Honey Board, there is no exact definition for raw honey. A honey label that says "untreated" or "unpasteurized" may be an indication, but not a guarantee that the honey is raw. Obviously, any honey labelled pasteurized is not raw. Don't be fooled by words like "natural" or "pure;" they mean nothing in regards to honey processing.

Many beekeepers will say that they consider honey raw only if it has not been heated above 105 degrees Fahrenheit.

Once processing heat exceeds 105 degrees, the consistency of raw honey changes along with the taste. Raw honey is smooth and creamy, can be found in liquid form, and has no aftertaste, while highly processed honey often has a somewhat smoky aftertaste.

Raw honey is obtained by extraction, settling or straining, and contains both pollen and small wax particles. This purest form of honey is alkalinizing and does not ferment in the stomach. It also contains amylase, an enzyme that helps break down foods containing starch.

To be sure that the honey you are purchasing is raw, it is best to get it from a local beekeeper who will tell you how the honey was obtained. The very best raw honey will also be organic - beekeepers must adhere to very strict regulations in order to be certified organic.

Strained honey: Also known as filtered honey, strained honey is honey that has been filtered to remove particles, but not pollen, prior to packaging.

Micro-filtered honey: When honey is micro or ultra-filtered, all particles, including the beneficial pollen, are removed and the honey is very clear. This honey can be stored for long periods of time. Be especially leery of ultra-filtered honey that has added sugar - this is sometimes the case - just read the label very carefully.

Pasteurized: Pasteurized honey is heated to increase shelf life and prevent crystallization. However, when honey is heated to a high temperature of 161 degrees Fahrenheit or higher, many of its beneficial properties are compromised.

Liquid honey: To get liquid honey, extractions are made in the comb so that the honey flows out. It can also be extracted by straining or centrifugation. This type of honey is sold widely throughout the United States.

Comb honey: A honeycomb is the natural storage compartment for honey created by honey bees. Comb honey is made of beeswax , which is made from nectar. It is a very pure form of honey, and was the original form of honey before extraction tools were invented. Comb honey is usually eaten as an appetizer, or can be spread or dunked in teas.

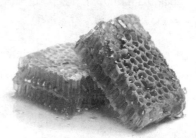

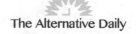

The Alternative Daily

Fact: Honey is the ONLY food produced by insects that humans can eat.

Cream honey: This honey is made by blending nine parts liquid honey with one part granulated honey. The mixture is stored until it becomes firm. Many people use this product as a spread like they would jams or jellies.

Chunk honey: This is just a mixture of comb and liquid honey, and is also called liquid-cut comb combination.

Naturally crystallized honey: The glucose in this honey is naturally in a crystallized state.

Testing Your Honey

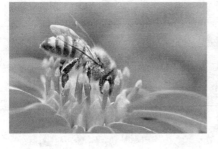

Most grocery store honey is loaded with cane sugar, corn syrup, invert sugar and water. To be sure that you are getting the best honey, here are two tests that you can perform:

Water dissolving test: Real honey will not dissolve readily in water, but adulterated honey will. Combine one tablespoon of honey and one cup of water and stir to test for authenticity.

Flame test: If water has been added to honey it will not burn. Place a cotton wick in a dollop of the honey and light it - pure honey will burn.

Worried about crystallization? Don't be...all honey will crystallize over time - it is actually a very good sign that the honey is raw. To re-liquify, all you have to do is gently heat the honey jar in warm water until it becomes liquid again - stir a bit and put back in the warm water if needed. There are some honeys that will not crystallize because they have very low glucose levels, including sourwood, honeydew, black locust-acacia, sunflower, sage and tupelo.

Other Products From the Hive

Beeswax

Used at one time as currency, beeswax is noted as the second most important product from the beehive. Worker bees have glands on their abdomens that produce wax scales for the colony. When more wax is needed for the expanding hive, bees generally aged 14 to 18 days gorge on honey and cluster together to raise their body temperature. After this, they make wax slivers. It takes a whopping 6 to 10 pounds of honey and 33,000 worker bee hours to produce 1 pound of wax, which contains about 450,000 wax slivers or scales and can hold about 22 pounds of honey.

Beeswax has been used since ancient times medicinally, and farmers in France even used it to pay their taxes in the 1300s. Beeswax is used around the world today for cosmetics, lubricants, candle making, inks, paints, electronics and more. In addition, beeswax is also recycled and put back into the honey industry - used for new honeycombs and queen cell cups.

Propolis

Propolis is also known as "bee glue," and is used to attach the combs to the tops and sides of hives, fill in cracks in the hive and embalm intruders. It is made up of a combination of plant resins, beeswax, balm, pollen and hive debris.

This sticky residue has been used medicinally since before 350 BC, mostly on wounds but also as a remedy for ailments including cancer, acne, itching, tuberculosis and osteoporosis. Propolis is used today to make chewing gum, creams and ointments, and is being investigated for use as a dental sealant and tooth enamel hardener. Some recent studies show that propolis may hold some promise for the treatment of burns, wounds, infections, dental pain and inflammatory conditions.

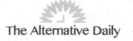

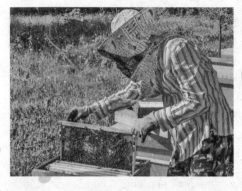

Brood

Selling of honey bee queens and worker bees is a special type of beekeeping that is highly lucrative. Worker bees are sold mostly in 3 lb packages that contain up to 10,000 bees. Queens are usually sold for more because of specific genetic origin or because they have desirable attributes. Queens are used by beekeepers to re-queen existing colonies where original queens may have been lost or are ill. Beekeepers can also expand their business by purchasing additional queens.

Pollen

Bee pollen is the male seed of a flower blossom, collected by honey bees and combined with the insects' digestive enzymes. It's a mixture of sticky pollen granules that can contain up to five million pollen spores each.

Raved about by many as a perfect superfood, bee pollen is considered one of nature's most complete foods when it comes to nourishment, containing nearly all nutrients humans need to thrive, including protein.

In fact, it's made up of 40 percent protein, with about half in the form of free amino acids that are ready to be used directly by the body. It's even richer in protein than any animal source and contains more amino acids than beef, eggs or cheese of equal weight. And, because it's so highly assimilable, it's an excellent source for meeting one's protein needs.

Of course this near-miracle food is nothing new — it may be one of the oldest foods on the planet, with bees and flowers evolving around the same time, roughly 150 million years ago. Bee pollen has been used for medicinal purposes for centuries, written about in many ancient records, and described by the ancient Egyptians as "life giving dust."

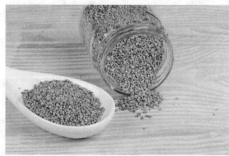

Bee pollen is rich in minerals, beneficial fatty acids, carotenoids and bioflavonoids which are antiviral and antibacterial, as well as essential vitamins, including B-complex and folic acid. Bee pollen is the only plant source that contains the important vitamin B12.

Bee venom

Although bee venom sounds like something you would want to avoid, scientists say that bee venom (and venom from snakes and scorpions) contains proteins and peptides that can be the source of valuable therapeutic compounds. Medicines derived from toxic venoms may have benefits in a wide range of diseases.

Bee venom therapy, also known as "apitherapy," involves the direct application of bee venom via injection into the skin. This unusual therapy may be beneficial for people suffering from arthritis, asthma, hearing loss, premenstrual syndrome, high blood pressure and multiple sclerosis.

Royal jelly

Even though the word "jelly" is incorporated into the name of this powerful superfood, royal jelly is a far cry from the sweet stuff you spread on toast. Rather, this potent jelly-like substance is secreted from the glands of worker bees in order to feed the queen bee and her larvae.

This often bitter-tasting substance is a combination of 60-70 percent water, 12-15 percent protein, 10-16 percent sugar, 3-6 percent fat and 2-3 percent vitamins, salt and amino acids. The specific combination is dependent on geography and climate.

In a typical bee colony, all bees start out as unisex larvae and develop into one of three roles: worker bees, drones or queen bees. All larvae begin their lives consuming the nutrient-rich royal jelly.

A typical worker bee or drone will be cut off from the premium royal jelly supply within a few days, and will enjoy an average lifespan of three to four months. Queen bees, however, continue their royal jelly diet and can live for as long as seven years.

Humans who have studied the development and differentiation of bees in the hive recognize that the key to the queen bee's longevity must be in her royal jelly-rich diet. This milky, jelly-like substance has been studied extensively for its effects on human health, specifically as a means of both preventing and treating diabetes.

While royal jelly exhibits promise in the realm of diabetes treatment, other research has found it to have bone-building effects in females, as well as being helpful in easing the symptoms of menopause. Early research has also pointed at anticancer, anti-inflammatory and energy-enhancing properties.

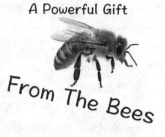

A Powerful Gift

From The Bees

You can find royal jelly in most health food stores, often in either pill or capsule form, as a powder or in its natural state (often frozen). Individuals with bee allergies should be especially careful when taking royal jelly, and those taking blood thinning medication like coumadin should avoid royal jelly as it is known to interfere with this medication and can result in increased bleeding or bruising.

> " *If the bee disappeared off the surface of the globe, then man would only have four years of life left.* "
> ~ Albert Einstein

The Plight of the Honey Bees

It would be remiss to write a book about honey without some mention of the current state of the honey bee. After all, the health of the honey bee population is directly related not only to honey production, but also to the world's food supply.

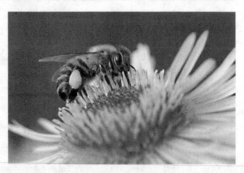

As you put your honey into your tea this morning, did it cross your mind that the bees that produce this wonderful, sweet treat are rapidly disappearing without a trace?

The honeybee population of our planet has been on a steady decline since the 1940s. In fact, in the 40's it was estimated that there were over 5 million honeybees in America, while today it is thought that there remain a scant 2.5 million. In the winter of 2012/2013, there was a 30 percent loss in honeybee colonies, which is the highest recorded loss in recent history.

Commonly referred to as colony collapse disorder (CCD), the disappearance of the bees is somewhat stumping researchers, who are scurrying to identify the problem and remedy the situation.

Everything from pathogens to parasites, environmental stressors to management stressors, are being reviewed in an effort to understand what is going on. At this point in time, there is no firm agreement as to why we seem to be losing our bees.

While lending a sympathetic ear to this tragic occurrence is a good place to start, it should not stop there. Even if you don't enjoy the sweet goodness of honey, the implications of losing honeybees is much further-reaching.

When you sit down at the dinner table, it is important to understand that one out of every three bites of food you put into your mouth comes from plants that have been pollinated by bees. Without bees, one third of all of our food would be gone. Bees contribute over 44 billion dollars a year to the United States economy.

To demonstrate the severity of the problem and to raise awareness, Whole Foods Market partnered with a nonprofit group called Xerces Society in a campaign labelled "Share the Buzz." To bring the point home, one Whole Foods store actually removed all produce that relies on bee pollination from their store shelves. Seeing the empty produce sections really created a visual impact for customers.

Over 237 of the 453 products in the store were removed. Among those gone were apples, bok choy, green onions, kale, leeks, limes, lemons, mangos, broc-

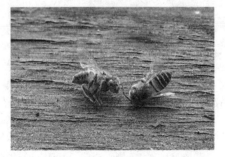

coli, summer squash, carrots, honeydew, cauliflower, cucumbers and celery. All of these foods and more are entirely dependent on bees.

More than 85 percent of the Earth's food system relies on pollinators to exist. Many of these foods are ones that provide us with the most nutrition, which makes matters much worse. We can all do without a toasted pastry, but if our fruits and veggies disappear, the health and economic implications will be vast.

What can be done?

While you may feel helpless when it comes to assisting bees, there is actually quite a bit that you can do. The first is to understand what is happening and commit to making a difference. Organizations such as the Xerces Society help farmers create wildflower habitats for bees and adopt less aggressive, less pesticide-intensive practices.

Beekeepers, concerned citizens and advocacy groups such as the Natural Resource Defence Council are begging for a stop to the use of dangerous pesticides called neonicotinoids. These chemicals are thought to be causing the bees to demonstrate the same symptoms that humans have with Parkinson's and Alzheimer's disease.

Just making this difference alone can do a great deal to create desirable habitats for bees. We can help save the bees and our food in other ways, as well. Adopting natural methods of running our homes and our gardens without the use of toxic pesticides is a start. Buying organic also supports the pollinators.

Planting bee-friendly flowers and fruits will help to provide habitats for the bees, and we can also shop in places where we see "Share the Buzz" signs.

Fact: It takes one ounce of honey to fuel a bee's flight around the world.

Good news… While the use of an insecticide class known as neonicotinoids is still widespread in the United States, some cities are taking action on a local level and banning their use, in an effort to both protect bee populations and the environment as a whole.

In June of this year, the city of Spokane, Washington banned the use of neonicotinoids within its borders. In 2013, Eugene, Oregon became the first city to enact such a ban.

These communities are responding to the severity of worldwide colony collapse disorder – the mass death of honeybees around the globe – and the growing scientific associations between this phenomenon and neonicotinoid insecticide use.

A recent review of 800 studies concluded that neonicotinoid use is connected to the mass deaths of insects, including bees and other pollinators. While not the only factor at play, the researchers state that they are playing a major role. According to Dr. Jean-Marc Bonmatin, one of the study's lead authors, "we are witnessing a threat to the productivity of our natural and farmed environment

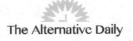

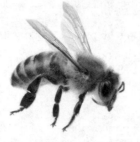

equivalent to that posed by organophos-phates or DDT."

The United Kingdom branch of the Pesticide Action Network (PAN) asserts, "neonicotinoids, especially seed treatments of imidacloprid and clothianidin on arable crops, have become of increasing concern to beekeepers and bee researchers in recent years with many of them suspecting that they may be connected to current bee declines."

Because of these concerns, the European Union began a two-year ban on three different neonicotinoids, imidacloprid, clothianidin and thiamethoxam, in 2013. The United States Environmental Protection Agency is reportedly "carefully watching" to see how this ban unfolds, and what results it produces.

Spokane, Washington, however, does not wish to wait for the federal government to determine how much damage these insecticides are doing. On the recent ban, City Council President Ben Stuckart stated, "this ordinance simply says Spokane prioritizes the protection of our food supply over the ornamental use of pesticides."

We hope that other communities take the examples of Spokane and Eugene to heart, and take a serious look at whether using these dangerous insecticides is worth the risk.

PART I *Honey for Health*

There are mountains of scientific research and clinical studies related to the medicinal properties of honey. A simple search on PubMed using the search term "honey" yields over 7,000 scientific papers dating back to 1884. The scientific and medical research community has invested heavily into understanding honey's remarkable therapeutic value. Unfortunately, much of this vast literature has gone largely unnoticed.

Below you will find summaries of the therapeutic uses of honey for a wide range of medical conditions. Each section is based on a body system, and you'll find information about how honey has been used therapeutically for medical conditions within that system. At the end of each section, you'll find practical applications for home use.

Skin Health

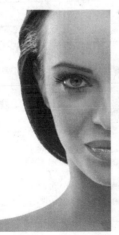

The skin is the body's largest and fastest-growing organ. Skin is the protective coat that keeps us warm when it is cold, cool when it is hot and keeps all of our inside parts inside, where they should be. It also keeps stuff like germs and water out.

Dermatology is a distinct medical specialty, concerned with the many illnesses and conditions that affect the skin. Dermatology is also the area where the therapeutic effects of honey have been the most widely studied. There are many illnesses, infections, and afflictions that can impact the skin

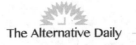

and cause everything from minor irritation to serious life threatening illness. Honey has repeatedly been proven to be a safe, effective and valuable tool in in keeping skin healthy, and looking and feeling great.

Seborrheic dermatitis: A common inflammatory condition that causes yellow and flaking skin, mostly in oily areas including on the face, in the ear and nose and on the scalp. It is also known as "cradle cap" when it occurs in infants. Although the exact cause is not known, it is thought that a weakened immune, endocrine or nervous system, or a yeast known as Malassezia, may play a part.

A study published in the European Journal of Medical Research looked at the effectiveness of raw honey in relieving seborrheic dermatitis and dandruff. Thirty participants suffering from seborrheic dermatitis and dandruff applied a mixture of 90 percent raw honey diluted in warm water to lesions every other day for four weeks. Those participants who showed improvement were included in a six month study where half were treated with topical honey weekly, and half served as a control group.

Researchers found those receiving the honey therapy had reduced itching and scaling within one week. At the two week mark, skin lesions healed completely and participants noted less hair loss. None of the participants who received a weekly application of honey had a relapse, while 12 out of 15 in the control group did. It was concluded that "crude honey could markedly improve seborrheic dermatitis and associated hair loss and prevent relapse when applied weekly."

In addition to making suggestions about dietary improvements and adding nutritional supplements like omega-3 fatty acids that can improve the general health of the skin, I recommend that patients with dandruff and seborrheic dermatitis use a topical application of diluted raw honey. I recommend making a paste using 90 percent raw honey and 10 percent warm water, just like what was done in the research. This paste should be applied to the affected areas, left on for three hours and then rinsed off. Do this treatment every other day for one month.

Atopic dermatitis (eczema): This is one of the most common skin conditions, and one of the most irritating. Eczema causes skin to be itchy and red, and repeated scratching often leads to thickening called lichenification. Eczematous areas are very prone to infection, which adds insult to injury. Although common in children, it can occur at any age and tends to be chronic with periodic flare-ups. Eczema is an allergic condition at its core, although the exact cause or trigger is often very difficult to pin down. There is also likely a genetic component that increases individual susceptibility, and there is mounting evidence our modern, "hyper-sanitary" environment may also contribute to an increased risk of eczema.

Researchers investigated the effects of a mixture of honey, olive oil and beeswax in a 1:1:1 ratio on patients who had atopic dermatitis. Twenty-one of the patients had no prior treatment before the honey mixture, and eleven used a topical corticosteroid cream before the trial.

Those participants who had received no prior treatment applied the honey mixture to affected areas on one side of their body and Vaseline to the affected areas on the other side of their body. This treatment was repeated three times a day for two weeks.

Those participants who were using the medicated cream prior to the trial applied a mixture of the cream and honey to one side of the body and a Vaseline and corticosteroid cream mixture to the other side. After the trial, patients were assessed for common eczema symptoms including skin thickening, redness, scaling, itching and oozing.

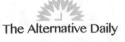

Eighty percent of those who had not used steroid creams before the trial had significant improvement with the honey mixture, and almost half of the patients who used the steroid cream before the trial did not have a worsening of symptoms when the steroid cream was replaced by the mixture of cream that contained three parts honey mixture and one part corticosteroids.

Honey can be used both internally and topically for this stubborn, itchy dermatitis. I advise eczema patients to add locally-produced raw honey to their diet, up to two tablespoons per day… usually added to herbal tea. Honey can be used topically for eczema as well. There are many commercially available honey-containing creams and ointments, but they are also really easy to make at home. Here's the recipe I give out to my patients:

Ingredients:

- One ounce raw honey (preferably Manuka)
- One ounce olive oil
- One ounce beeswax (a chunk about the size of an ice cube)

Instructions:

1. Melt the beeswax slowly in a saucepan.
2. Remove from heat and add the honey and olive oil.
3. While the mixture is still warm, add to a jar with an airtight lid.
4. Store in the refrigerator for up to three months.
5. Apply to affected areas up to three times per day.

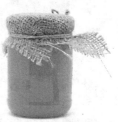

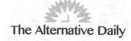

Tinea versicolor: This is a very common skin condition, especially in tropical and subtropical areas of the world. Tinea versicolor is a fungal infection that produces a rash of variable colors which typically become more prominent as the skin tans, hence its name, "versicolor." In addition to the skin discoloration, tinea versicolor can also cause a sharp itching sensation. It is considered a minimally contagious infection.

A 2004 study out of Dubai Specialized Medical Center and Medical Research Laboratories investigated using honey as an alternative treatment for tinea versicolor. Thirty-seven patients used a mixture of one-part honey, one-part beeswax and one part olive oil to treat the fungal infection. The mixture was applied to lesions three times a day for four weeks. Over 70 percent of those treated with the honey mixture experienced healing from the condition.

In another study, 61 high school students with tinea versicolor were instructed to apply a thin coating of pure honey (collected from a 6 month old beehive) to affected areas twice a day for 30 days. At the end of the study period, a 98.36 percent cure rate was observed.

I have found that the same recipe used for eczema (honey/beeswax/olive oil in a 1:1:1 ratio) can also be applied to tinea versicolor. This mixture can be alone or in addition to other treatments like selenium sulfide applications.

Intertrigo: This is an infection and inflammation of the skin folds in areas such as the armpits, genital area, and beneath the breasts and the abdomen. It is a painful, bright red rash that often has a discharge with a foul odor and cracked, crusty or oozing skin.

Thirty-one patients with symmetrical intertrigo in skin folds were instructed to use a routine therapy of zinc oxide on one side of their body and honey as a barrier

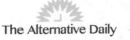

cream on the other side of their body. The study period lasted 21 days, and at the end, both therapies appeared to be effective, although the honey actually reduced patient itching complaints more than the zinc oxide. It was determined that honey barrier cream is a suitable alternative treatment for intertrigo, and also promotes patient comfort.

I advise patients with this rash within skin folds to use topical honey directly. There are some commercially available products, such as MediHoney barrier cream, which have been used in research, but manuka honey straight from the jar seems to work just as well.

Diaper rash: Anyone who has had children has probably experienced diaper rash, also known as "napkin rash" (they call diapers napkins or "nappies" in the UK). This painful condition often occurs as a reaction to a new food, diaper chafing, a yeast infection or irritation from urine.

A New Zealand study investigated using topical pharmaceutical-grade kanuka honey in place of traditional barrier cream for treatment of redness, itching and inflammation. The kanuka tree (Kunzea ericoides) is native to New Zealand and is similar in appearance to the manuka shrub. It has been found that kanuka honey has greater anti-inflammatory capability than manuka. Participants were instructed to apply a thin layer of honey in the same fashion as they would barrier cream. Researchers found that compliance was high and that symptoms were improved in a similar fashion to using barrier cream.

Whether diaper rash is caused by simple irritation or is complicated by infection (often yeast), topical honey can be very helpful. I recommend that parents add equal parts of honey to their favorite diaper cream and apply directly to the rash at each diaper change.

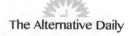

Herpes simplex: This common viral infection results in cold sores or fever blisters. Even when sores are not visible, this condition is contagious, spreads easily and can be highly uncomfortable.

In a study, sixteen adults who had frequent labial and genital herpes attacks used honey to treat one attack and a common prescription cream, Acyclovir, to treat another. The honey provided significantly better results than the cream. For labial herpes, the mean healing time was forty-three percent better, and for genital herpes it was fifty-nine percent better than the prescription cream.

The honey reduced pain and crusting and caused no side effects, while the cream caused local itching in three subjects.

Pain and crusting were also significantly reduced with the honey compared to the drug. Two cases of labial herpes and one case of genital herpes remitted completely with the honey treatment, whereas none remitted while using Acyclovir.

The researchers concluded, "topical honey application is safe and effective in the management of the signs and symptoms of recurrent lesions from labial and genital herpes."

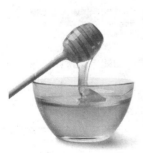

There are many natural and nutritional recommendations that I advise to patients with recurrent herpes outbreaks on the lips (cold sores) or in the genital area. With respect to the use of honey, I recommend that they do exactly what was done in the research studies. This protocol involves pressing honey-soaked gauze firmly on the lesions for 15 minutes four times per day. Make sure to use new gauze each time.

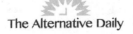

Staphylococcus aureus: Many people have this bacteria on their skin and in their noses and it never causes a problem. However, when the skin is broken, the bacteria can enter and cause a host of issues. Staph bacteria can spread through contaminated surfaces or between people.

Manuka honey can be applied directly to superficial infections or be added to a bandage or wound dressing. Any skin infection that is rapidly spreading or causes a fever needs immediate medical attention.

Candida albicans: This condition, commonly known as a yeast infection, is caused by the overgrowth of a common organism called Candida albicans. Although candida is a normal inhabitant of multiple sites in and on our bodies, its growth is normally kept in check by our own immune system and other beneficial microorganisms. Overgrowth of yeast can affect the skin, genitals, throat, mouth and blood. Certain medications (especially antibiotics) and conditions like diabetes can cause this naturally-occurring yeast to overgrow.

It always surprises patients when I suggest that honey can be useful in the treatment of yeast infections. Many patients with chronic or recurrent problems with yeast have been advised to follow very low carbohydrate diets and avoid all sugars, including honey. However, there have in fact been many studies that demonstrate that honey is a safe, effective, broad spectrum antifungal agent. Raw or manuka honey can be applied directly to candida infections two to three times per day.

Pressure ulcers: Also known as bedsores, these uncomfortable sores on the skin can be caused by any number of things, including lying in bed or sitting in a wheelchair. These sore spots can also result from diabetes and other vascular diseases.

In a research study, two groups, each with pressure ulcers, were studied. One group received a honey dressing while the other was treated with ethoxy-diaminoacridine plus nitrofurazone dressings. After the five-week study period was up, the group who received the honey dressings experienced four times the rate of healing as the group that received the medicated dressings.

If you or a loved one has a deep pressure ulcer, consider applying a honey-soaked gauze pad to the wound and covering with a second semipermeable bandage to prevent leakage.

Surgical wounds: Surgical wounds are made by using a cutting instrument during a medical procedure. Although these incisions are made in a sterile environment, they can sometimes be hard to heal or become infected.

Studies have shown honey to be effective in the treatment of infected surgical wounds. Researchers found that unboiled honey accelerated wound healing when applied topically - this they attributed to its hydrogen peroxide-producing effect, and its antimicrobial and hygroscopic properties.

I advise my patients with surgical wounds to begin using topical raw manuka honey dressings as soon as they can after surgery. Honey can be applied directly to the surgical wound or can be added to a bandage or wound dressing. Fresh honey should be used with each dressing change, at least once per day.

Skin grafts: A skin graft is a type of graft surgery involving the transplantation of skin, often used to treat burns or other serious skin trauma.

In 2003, a study published in the journal Dermatologic Surgery looked at the use of honey in healing a split-thickness skin graft donor site. Study leaders concluded that using gauzes impregnated with honey is a safe and practical application, and a good alternative to traditional skin graft dressings material for healing. In the study, part of the group received the honey bandages while the others received paraffin gauzes, saline-soaked gauzes and hydrocolloid dressings. Those that received the honey dressings had faster epithelization time and less pain than the others.

In my practice, I do not tend to see skin grafts until long after they are healed. That said, there is some very compelling literature that suggest that honey can be safely and effectively used in the fixation and healing of skin graft sites. Only medical grade honey preparations should be used for this purpose.

Burns: Heat, electricity, chemicals, radiation and chemicals can cause serious injury to the skin. Deep or very widespread burns can leave skin very vulnerable to bacterial infection, which may increase the risk of sepsis.

Honey has proven itself to be a highly effective treatment in the case of burns. Research out of New Zealand points to the effectiveness of manuka honey in treating burns. The Journal of Cutaneous and Aesthetic Surgery published a paper based on an analysis comparing the use of medicated dressings (Silver Sulfadiazine) with honey dressings over a five-year period. The analysis involved 108 patients with first and second degree burns over less than 50 percent of their bodies. Of the patients, 57 received the medicated bandages and 51 the honey dressings.

When burn healing time was compared, those patients with the honey dressings healed in an average of 18.16 days, while those with the medicated bandages healed in 32.68 days. In addition, the wounds of patients treated with the honey bandages became sterile in less than 7 days, while wounds of patients treated with the medicated bandages became sterile in 21 days.

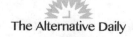

Researchers concluded that the honey dressings made wounds sterile in a shorter time period and also improved healing time.

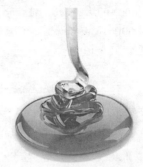

For superficial burns that can be treated at home, honey can be very effective at improving healing and decreasing the risk of infection. Apply raw honey directly to the burn three times per day. Alternatively, use a bandage soaked in honey or the homemade honey/beeswax/olive oil recipe as a burn cream.

Wound healing: There are many things that can impact wound healing time, including severity, promptness and type of medical care and how sterile the wound is kept.

Hospitals all over the world are now using active manuka honey alongside conventional medication to treat a number of conditions, with wound healing topping the list. During the Civil War, honey was applied liberally to the wounds of soldiers, and today, scientists are finding out that manuka honey has the ability to stop dangerous infections in their tracks.

Professor Elizabeth Harry, from the University of Technology, Sydney, reported in the journal PLOS ONE that manuka is the best honey for stopping bacterial infections and wounds. In addition, manuka honey has been shown effective in the treatment of eczema, burns, dermatitis and abscesses.

A study conducted in 1992 showed that manuka honey sped healing after caesarean sections. The Journal of Lower Extremity Wounds found positive findings on honey in wound care reported from 17 randomized control trials including more than 1,965 participants, as well as from 16 trials involving wounds on over 500 experimental animals.

Six years ago, the FDA authorized the very first honey-based medical product for use in America. Derma Sciences uses manuka honey for their Medihoney burn and wound dressings, which you can find online and in medical supply stores.

Raw honey can be applied to a Band-Aid, or onto a gauze pad, and applied directly to the site. Dressings or bandages should be changed at least every 24 hours.

Endocrine and Metabolic Systems

The endocrine system is the factory, the warehouse and the shipping department for hormones. Hormones are produced by a network of glands, which secrete them directly into the bloodstream. Endocrine hormones have an influence on virtually all bodily functions, including important effects on metabolism. Collectively, the endocrine system regulates every cell and organ in the body, controlling such functions as metabolism, sexual functions, mood, cell growth and development.

The term "metabolism" refers to a series of chemical reactions used to produce cellular energy by burning fuel. There are thousands of metabolic reactions that occur constantly within our cells to keep them vital and functioning optimally.

There are a number of disorders that can affect the endocrine and metabolic systems and lead to a variety of dysfunctions, diseases and medical conditions.

Fasting blood sugar levels in diabetics: Diabetes is a common metabolic ailment that is caused by a disorder in the regulation and control of blood sugar.

People who have diabetes have elevated glucose, also called hyperglycemia or high blood sugar.

Although honey is sweet, it has a fairly low glycemic index. The natural sugars in honey have a "slow-release" effect, which means it does not cause the sharp peak in blood sugar that other sweet substances (like refined sugar) do. The sugars in honey are therefore more slowly absorbed and metabolized. Despite its sweetness, honey will not cause blood sugar levels to spike as high or as fast as other high-sugar foods.

In a study conducted on healthy, diabetic patients who also were hyperlipidemic, honey had the following impact:

Blood sugar levels were not elevated to the same extent as with glucose and sucrose.

- Lowered bad cholesterol and raised good cholesterol.
- Reduced C-reactive protein - a marker for inflammation.
- Lowered homocysteine - another blood indicator of disease.

Even the biggest supporters of the medicinal uses of honey have been surprised at the research on honey and diabetes. Based on studies in rodents that have demonstrated improvements in several measures of diabetes complications, researchers have begun to test the effects of honey consumption on humans with diabetes as well. Although it is generally wise for diabetics to avoid sugar and sweets, these early studies have suggested that there may be an exception to the rule when it comes to honey. It has been shown that honey has a lower glycemic effect than simple sugar. While it may seem completely crazy to suggest honey to someone with diabetes, I now tell my diabetic patients that they can use up to 1 tablespoon (about 20 grams) of honey per day.

> "Honey consumption (as compared to refined sugar or HFCS) leads directly to the formation of liver glycogen, thus stabilising blood sugar levels. Honey thereby reduces metabolic stress and improves fat metabolism and disposal, thus combating two of the key parameters of the metabolic syndrome, Type 2 Diabetes and obesity."

~Dr Ron Fessenden, *The Honey Revolution*

Homocysteine levels: Homocysteine is an amino acid which is a product of protein metabolism. When found in high concentrations, this product has been linked to an increase in the risk of heart attack and stroke. Elevated homocysteine levels may contribute to the formation of plaque and arterial wall damage. There is also some evidence to suggest that persons with elevated homocysteine levels may have up to twice the normal risk of developing Alzheimer's disease.

As mentioned above, honey appears to lower homocysteine levels, thereby reducing the risk of heart attack and stroke.

Although the general rule for lowering plasma homocysteine levels involves the use of B vitamins, there is also some limited evidence that honey can help as well. When patients have elevated homocysteine levels, I tell them that they can safely consume up to 40 grams (about two tablespoons) of honey per day.

Blood glucose control in Type 1 diabetes: Once known as juvenile diabetes or insulin-dependent diabetes, Type 1 diabetes is a chronic condition in which the pancreas fails to produce sufficient insulin. Insulin is the hormone that allows sugar (glucose) to leave the blood and enter the cells so the absence of insulin causes the blood sugar to rise while the cells are starving. This is why diabetes is sometimes referred to as "starving in the midst of plenty."

A review of scientific literature indicates that honey has a positive impact on the treatment of diabetes. Research findings reinforce the therapeutic prospects of using honey, or other potent antioxidants such as vitamin C or E, as an adjunct to standard anti-diabetic drugs in the management of diabetes mellitus.

The study authors wrote, "the beneficial effects of honey in diabetes might not only be limited to controlling glycemia but might also extend to improving the associated metabolic derangements in this complicated metabolic disorder."

I encourage my Type I diabetes patients to keep their diets as low-glycemic as possible. I also tell them that of all of the available sweeteners on the market, honey is the best choice.

Antioxidants in blood: Human blood has fascinated scientists, philosophers, artists and children for millennia. It is the source of all that nourishes us, as it carries oxygen, vitamins, minerals and proteins that are pumped through miles of vessels within our body. The quality of our blood is vital to all systems, and to our overall health and well-being. A low red blood cell count can cause fatigue, anemia and weakness. Healthy blood supports the immune system and protects us from infections and disease. Healthy blood contains high levels of antioxidant compounds, some of which are made internally and others that are consumed in the diet.

Antioxidants help to prevent oxidation… a common underlying cause of a wide variety of illnesses. There are many conditions that have been linked to low anti-oxidant levels and the resultant "oxidative stress." Diseases such as diabetes, hypertension, heart disease, Alzheimer's disease and cancer are on the rise. These conditions and many more are known to be associated with increased oxidative stress.

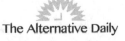

So, what are antioxidants? Antioxidants are natural substances that prevent or slow cell damage. When our blood cells and vessels contain high levels of anti-oxidants, this leads to decreased risks of a variety of diseases including cardio-vascular disease, diabetes, and cancer.

According to a report published in the journal Molecules in 2012:

> *Honey is a natural substance with many medicinal effects such as anti-bacterial, hepatoprotective, hypoglycemic, reproductive, antihyperten-sive and antioxidant effects.*

Antioxidants found in foods are a valuable nutritional resource. Fresh fruits and vegetables are the most commonly cited sources of antioxidants in food, but numerous research studies indicate that honey (especially dark honey) also contains potent antioxidants. Adding raw honey into one's diet (especially dark honey) can help keep antioxidant levels high in the bloodstream.

Immune System and Infections

The immune system is our department of defense, our intelligence agency, and our military. It is comprised of cells, tissues, and organs which work together as our primary defense against infectious organisms and other dangerous invaders. The immune system can recognize and attack these organisms before they cause us problems. There are a wide range of conditions that can impact the strength and agility of our immune system and when it is compromised, we invite in a host of dangerous organisms that can cause illness.

> *It may seem odd that straight exposure to pollen often triggers allergies but that exposure to pollen in the honey usually has the opposite effect...In honey the allergens are delivered in small, manageable doses and the effect over time is very much like that from undergoing a whole series of allergy immunology injections.*
>
> ~Thomas Leo Ogren, "Allergy-Free Gardening

Allergies: Millions of Americans suffer with allergies. There are hundreds of substances that can provoke allergic symptoms in susceptible individuals. Allergic triggers can be airborne (ie. pollen, dust or animal dander), foodborne (ie. peanuts or shellfish) or via skin exposure (ie. latex or poison ivy.) Allergy symptoms can vary from minor irritations to life threatening illness. There are many approaches to the treatment of allergy, by far the most common are pharmaceuticals. Both over-the-counter and prescription medications may help to un-stuff your sinuses, but they often come with a host of unpleasant side effects. Some antihistamines might leave you feeling groggy and foggy, others cause people to feel jittery and anxious. Beyond that is a long list of other potential adverse effects, including symptoms like altered taste and smell and possibly more serious issues such as female infertility. Non-drug approaches to allergy treatment are in high demand, and honey can really help.

A 2011 study published in the International Archives of Allergy and Immunology found that patients who were diagnosed with birch pollen allergy were able to reduce 60 percent of their allergy symptoms and decrease the number of days with severe symptoms by 70 percent by taking birch pollen honey pre-seasonally. This was a specialized honey that had tiny amounts of birch pollen added for an additional "desensitization" effect.

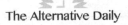

Thousands of people swear by this remedy, but buying just any honey off the grocery store shelf won't do the trick. It's got to be local honey, as bees produce it by traveling around local plants and gathering local pollen, which is what you're reacting to when you have allergies. By ingesting local honey, it helps to create immunity to those specific allergens in your area. Eat local honey all year round to derive the most benefits.

Locally-produced honey is one of my favorite treatments for seasonal allergies. It can improve markers and symptoms of immunity with people with allergies. I tell allergy patients to find a local beekeeper (they're often at farmers markets) and ask them for honey that was made during the season that they get allergies. Local, seasonal honey can then be consumed daily at doses of up to two tablespoons per day. I often suggest that the honey be added to a tea made with nettle (Urtica dioaca) leaf, which has additional anti-allergy benefits.

E. coli: While E. coli bacteria live in the intestines of healthy people and animals and most are quite harmless, some strains can cause severe stomach cramps, bloody diarrhea and vomiting. You can be exposed to E. coli from food or water that has been contaminated - especially raw vegetables or undercooked ground beef.

Studies have clearly demonstrated that honey inhibits the growth of E. coli in petri-dishes and in animal models of infection. Although I don't recommend using honey exclusively to treat this infection, it is reasonable to include herbals teas sweetened with honey as an adjunct to treatment for E. coli.

Fournier's gangrene: Although rare, this disease is life-threatening and is an infection in the genital area that normally impacts men. If the infection spreads to the blood, sepsis can occur and result in death.

First of all… I hope you never encounter this problem. It is a dreadful and dangerous urogenital infection. That said, a team of Turkish urologists have studied and published the results of their work using honey in addition to standard hospital care for this infection, and have demonstrated impressive results.

Antibiotic resistant superbugs: A troubling new report issued by the World Health Organization (WHO) sheds light on the severity of the rising global problem of antibiotic resistance, and cautions that if significant changes are not soon made, the world could be headed for a "post-antibiotic era," in which diseases that were once under control by modern medicine could threaten once again. Antibiotic resistance is, according to the CDC, a leading world health problem. Doctors first began to notice resistance problems almost a decade ago, when kids with middle-ear infections stopped responding to the drugs they were being given.

Penicillin has also become less effective over time, and a new strain of staph bacteria has arisen that does not respond to antibiotics at all. This makes honey an attractive option for treating wounds, burns and skin problems that could develop into serious infections.

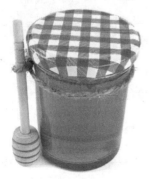

Dr. Ralf Schlothauer, PhD, the CEO of Comvita, New Zealand's largest supplier of medicinal manuka, explains that the UMF (Unique Manuka Factor) certification of manuka honey is a concentration of the individual antioxidant phenols that are in the honey. These phenols inhibit bacterial growth and promote healing. These antioxidants are not like synthetic antibiotics that promote the spread of antibiotic-resistant superbugs.

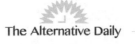

It is entirely clear that raw honey is an impressive antimicrobial agent against a broad spectrum of bacteria and other infectious organisms. When my patients have infections, including tough-to-treat infections like MRSA and other antibiotic-resistant organisms, I will include the internal and external use of raw manuka honey.

Eyes, Ears, Nose, Throat and Mouth

The eyes, ears, nose, throat and mouth are subject to a variety of painful conditions and infections. ENT (ear, nose and throat) infections are one of the most common reasons for visits to primary care physicians. It is common for physicians to use either antibiotics or prescription steroids to treat many of the problems that arise in the eyes, ears, nose and throat. Although pharmaceuticals do play an important role in the treatment of these problems, often, non-drug therapies including honey can be safe, effective alternatives.

Tonsillectomy: This is a procedure that removes the tonsil glands located on the back of the throat. These glands are often removed along with the adenoid glands. Pain following the surgery can vary between moderate and intense. I always try to help my patients avoid surgery whenever possible, including tonsillectomy. There are times though when the tonsils are such a problem that surgical removal is necessary. In those cases, honey after surgery is not only a sweet treat, but can actually help with recovery.

Researchers have found that postoperative honey administration reduced patient pain and need for analgesics. It was also noted that compared to analgesics, honey has negligible side effects.

I recommend that after tonsillectomy, patients take one teaspoon of honey every two to three hours while they are awake. It can be taken right off of a spoon, or diluted in about one ounce of warm water.

Fungal sinusitis: The sinuses are cavities within the skull that are warm, dark and moist. They make cozy little homes for microbes including fungi. Fungal infections can cause inflammation and pain in the sinuses, just like bacterial infections. Bacterial sinusitis is most commonly treated with antibiotics and often a nasal steroid spray to reduce inflammation. Fungal infections require a totally different approach and can be difficult to treat, because these organisms are not killed by antibiotics and steroid nasal sprays can often make fungal infections worse. However, honey can help.

I recommend that sinusitis sufferers try making their own honey nasal spray. The recipe used in the studies is simply 50/50 raw manuka honey and saline, used as a nasal spray two to three times daily.

This solution can be prepared using store-bought saline (which can be purchased in a convenient nasal spray bottle) or be made at home using this recipe:

Simple Saline:

- ¼- ½ teaspoon of finely ground non-iodized salt
- ¼ teaspoon baking soda
- 1 cup distilled water

NOTE: Another really easy way to make saline is to buy the prepackaged packets of salt/baking soda that are used to prepare the solution for nasal irrigation. Simply add 1 packet to 1 cup of distilled water and you are good to go.

These packets are inexpensive, convenient, and can be found near the nasal sprays at any drugstore.

Allergic rhinitis (runny nose): Allergic rhinitis is an annoying and uncomfortable condition that is caused by an allergic inflammation in the nasal airways. Inflammation may result when pollen, dust or animal dander is inhaled by people with sensitive immune systems. As you've learned, good quality local honey actually contains pollen, often pollen derived from plants that cause seasonal allergies. Although it seems counter-intuitive to consume the pollen from the plants that you are allergic to, it seems that ingesting the pollen in honey can actually help in cases of pollen allergy. Immunologists are still working on why this might be; it's possible that the action of enzymes found in honey and the "low and slow" doses of pollen may help to improve immune tolerance in a similar way that allergy shots are known to work.

Allergic rhinitis and hayfever responds really well to honey both internally, and topically as a nasal spray. I advise seasonal allergy patients to consume local, seasonal raw honey at a dose of 1 tablespoon per day. I also suggest that they use a daily nasal spray made with equal parts honey and simple saline.

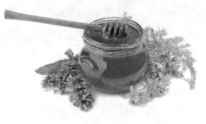

Meibomian gland dysfunction (MGD): MGD is thought to be the leading cause of dry eye syndrome. Meibomian glands are a special type of sebaceous gland located at the rim of the eyelid. This gland is responsible for making meibum, an oily substance that prevents evaporation of the eye's tear film.

Preliminary studies have suggested that eye drops made from sterilized manuka honey can be useful in treating dry eyes related to meibomian gland dysfunction. These drops must be sterile and prepared for ophthalmic use. Two or three drops are added to the lower lid three times per day.

Corneal erosions: Corneal erosions impact the cornea, the clear dome covering on the front of the eye. The cornea is comprised of five layers, and the outermost layer is called the epithelium. When this layer does not stay attached to the tissue below it can cause a corneal erosion. This condition is painful, and usually feels worst in the morning when waking up because the eyes tend to get dry at night.

There is some preliminary evidence that adding honey to usual care for corneal abrasions and erosions can be helpful in decreasing the potential for infection and speeding healing, as well as for helping to ensure that vision is preserved. Eye drops made with manuka honey are used for this purpose - these drops must be sterile and prepared for ophthalmic use.

Infections in the mouth: Bacteria and viruses can cause oral infections that impact the teeth, gums, palate, tongue, lips and the inside of the cheeks. Oral infections are very common. In fact, infections that cause tooth decay are the second most common infectious condition after the common cold.

Researchers in India have found that manuka honey worked just as well as commercial mouthwash, and better than chewing gum with xylitol, for reducing plaque levels. This they attribute to its outstanding antibacterial qualities. Manuka honey, taken orally, can help reduce gingivitis and keep the mouth healthy and free from harmful bacteria.

A variety of infections and irritations in the mouth can be successfully treated with honey. I typically recommend using undiluted raw honey at a dose of one teaspoon three to four times per day. Swish the honey around your mouth and over the irritated area, then swallow.

Pulmonary/Respiratory System

A breath of fresh air... sounds good, right? Well, that life-giving breath is the primary responsibility of your respiratory system. In medicine, we think of the respiratory tract in two parts. The "upper" respiratory tract includes the nose, nasal passages, sinuses and the pharynx and larynx, which are in the throat. The "lower" respiratory tract includes the trachea (or windpipe), the bronchi, and the lungs themselves. All of our cells require oxygen in order to function, and without it we would cease to exist. The pulmonary/respiratory system is responsible for ensuring that our cells get the fresh oxygen they need.

There are many conditions that can compromise the function of the respiratory tract, most commonly upper and lower respiratory infections. Honey can play a valuable role in managing upper and lower respiratory tract problems.

Respiratory infections and cough: Upper respiratory infections, also known as colds, impact the nose, throat, larynx and windpipe. Colds are often caused by a viral infection and can lead to runny nose, cough, sore throat and laryngitis. Lower respiratory infections involve the bronchial airway and the lungs.

For common coughs and colds, honey can act as both an antimicrobial agent and a cough suppressant. Use 1 teaspoon of raw honey every 3-4 hours. It can be given directly off the spoon or diluted in a little warm water or herbal tea. Ginger tea with honey and lemon is a family favorite. One teaspoon of honey straight off the spoon before bed can really help with nighttime coughs in kids.

For a lingering cough, consider the results of a fascinating new study, which tells us that a mixture of coffee and honey is equally, if not more, effective as a steroid cough syrup for silencing a persistent post-infectious cough (PPC).

A post-infectious cough is one that lasts for three to five weeks after a common cold or respiratory infection. This is the cough that keeps you up at night and interferes with your normal daily routine. A cough such as this can make you tired, irritable and is nothing short of very annoying. These coughs are commonly treated with antibiotics and/or steroids… neither of which are terribly effective.

The study mentioned above compared the effectiveness of a systemic steroid medication and honey plus coffee to treat this lingering cough. Ninety-seven adults who had PPC for at least three weeks were divided into three groups.

One group received a jam-like paste made from coffee and honey, another group received a steroid medication (prednisolone) and a third group received a non-steroidal cough syrup (guaifenesin). The pastes were made to be similar in texture and flavor so that the participants did not know what they were taking. They were instructed to dissolve their syrup in warm water and consume once every 8 hours for one week. Cough frequency was measured.

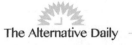

Study results clearly demonstrated that the group who took the coffee and honey mixture had the greatest decrease in cough frequency, and researchers noted that this combination was the best treatment choice for PPC.

According to the study authors: "Each year, billions of dollars are spent on controlling and trying to cure coughs while the real effect of cough medicines is not quite reliable. Even though PPC is reported to account for only 11–25% of all cases of chronic cough and it is not associated with disability and mortality, it can cause morbidity and is responsible for medical costs..."

This study adds to a rapidly growing body of biomedical research that indicates the power and potency of natural substances including spices, herbs, vitamins and foods. Not only are they being found to be equally as effective, but also superior in efficacy when compared to synthetic drugs – not to mention the fact that they are almost always less expensive!

The recipe used in the study is easy to prepare at home:

Honey/Coffee Cough Syrup:

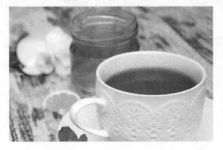

The recipe used in the study involved making a big batch of syrup using 500 grams of honey and 70 grams of instant coffee mixed together. Then, one tablespoon of this pasty syrup was dissolved into one cup of water every 8 hours for one week.

This translates to about 1.5 cups of honey mixed with about ¾ cup of instant coffee.

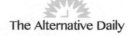

If you choose to make a big batch like they did in the study, then use 1 table-spoon of this mixture per cup of water. If you want to make individual doses to dissolve into water one cup a at time, use 1 tablespoon of honey to 1.5 teaspoons of instant coffee.

Gastrointestinal System

The gastrointestinal (GI) tract is essentially a long tube that is responsible for digestion, absorption and elimination. Foods are broken down into nutrients that can can be absorbed to support life, and the leftovers get eliminated. The GI tract is commonly divided into two sections. The upper GI tract includes the esophagus, stomach, and the upper part of the small intestine called the duodenum. The lower GI tract includes the rest of the small intestine and the entire length of the large intestine. Because of its role as the entry point for food and nutrition, problems within the GI tract can often be at the "root" of many different medical problems that cause symptoms both inside and outside of the GI system itself.

Acid reflux disease: Although there is minimal published scientific data to support the use of honey in the treatment of acid reflux, it is a widely used "folk" remedy for heartburn. I have seen many patients who tell me that honey helps them feel better from intermittent heartburn symptoms. I don't use honey alone to treat this illness because there are many very useful natural medicine strate-gies to help improve acid reflux, but I do believe that honey is a reasonable part of a natural treatment plan for heartburn.

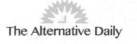

Candida overgrowth: Candida is a species of yeast. It is a part of the normal flora, which refers to the massive ecosystem of microbes that live inside and outside of our bodies. Candia lives on our skin, and is a resident in the community of organisms that inhabit the gastrointestinal tract. Everyone has a small amount of yeast living in their mouth and intestines.

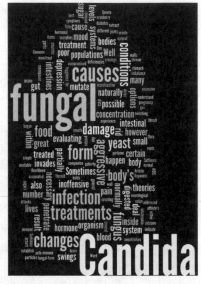

Small amounts of candida are normal and don't cause any problems. In fact, it may even play a role in digestion and nutrient absorption. Problems arise when candida populations overgrow and overpopulate… this is known as a yeast infection or candida overgrowth. This condition often results from overuse of antibiotics which kill off the "good bugs" which help to compete with the yeast for territory. When those good bugs are killed, yeast can flourish. Overgrowth of yeast can set the stage for a wide range of subsequent medical problems, so it is important to use safe and effective strategies to prevent and treat this problem.

Many patients who have overgrowth of intestinal yeast (candida) are advised to strictly avoid all sugar, sweets and simple carbohydrates, including honey. These diets can be very helpful, but they are also very restrictive and difficult to follow. Although honey may not be a stand-alone treatment for intestinal yeast, patients are always thrilled to find out that the inclusion of honey into an anti-candida diet

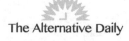

The Alternative Daily

is safe and should not interfere with their efforts to eradicate candida. Honey is the sweetener of choice for people with intestinal yeast overgrowth… up to 2 teaspoons per day are usually fine.

Inflammatory bowel disorders: The most common inflammatory bowel disorders (IBD) are ulcerative colitis and Crohn's disease. Both are serious illnesses that require medical attention. Ulcerative colitis is a chronic recurrent disease involving the colon, which causes inflammation and bleeding. Crohn's disease is also a chronic recurrent disease, but may involve any portion of the gastrointestinal tract and usually causes patchy areas of inflammation.

The exact cause of these conditions is not clear, but there appear to be multiple possible triggers. Genetic influences, autoimmune features, infections, lifestyle factors, stress and diet/nutrition may all play a role.

Inflammatory bowel disease is a serious illness, and most of my patients require a comprehensive "integrative" approach that includes the use of both conventional and naturopathic medicine.

There are many factors to consider when developing a treatment strategy for IBD, but honey can play a role. Based on animal research and on my own clinical experience, honey is the sweetener of choice for patients with ulcerative colitis and Crohn's disease. I suggest up to 1 tablespoon two times per day.

Cancer: Cancer is one of the most feared conditions in medicine. Thousands of medical visits occur every day from individuals who are worried that they might have cancer. Most of them simply need reassurance from a doctor, but unfortunately, sometimes they're right, and they need more than just reassurance. There are well over 100 different types of cancer, which can affect virtually every cell type. Damaged cells divide uncontrollably to form masses called tumors, which

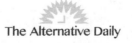

The Alternative Daily

can grow and spread and impair the function of the system that they invade. It is widely known that eating well, avoiding carcinogenic exposures (like tobacco smoke), and regular physical activity can reduce the risk of cancer substantially. And the old adage is certainly true when it comes to cancer: "an ounce of prevention is worth a pound of cure."

Honey has been the subject of significant research in the field of oncology. Much of this research is "in-vitro" work... studies on cancer cells in a petri dish or test tube in a laboratory setting. There are also some early animal studies and a fair amount of research using honey to help decrease the adverse effects of a number of different conventional cancer treatments.

Colon cancer: There is evidence that honey plus ginger can have an anti-cancer effect on colon cancer cells in-vitro. Although there is no reliable evidence demonstrating that this effect remains true in human clinical trials, it is reasonable to include honey as the sweetener of choice in patients with colon cancer.

Leukemia: In-vitro and animal research has demonstrated that honey has anti-proliferative and apoptotic effects. This essentially means that it can inhibit the growth of leukemia cells. Although there is no reliable evidence demonstrating that this effect remains true in human clinical trials, it is reasonable to include honey as the sweetener of choice in patients with hematologic (tumors that affect blood, bone marrow and lymph nodes) malignancies like leukemia.

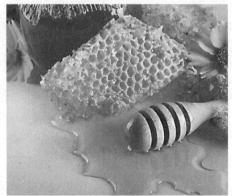

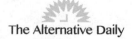

Radiation in head and neck cancers: One of the most unpleasant side effects of radiation therapy in head and neck cancers is a problem called mucositis, or inflammation of the mucous membranes in the mouth, nose or throat. There are conflicting reports of the value of topically-applied raw honey in this painful condition. There are other useful therapies to both treat and prevent this painful condition, but it is reasonable to include a direct topical honey application to the site of the radiation damage 2-3 times daily.

Breast cancer treatment: There is some laboratory and animal research that suggests that Tualang honey (from Malaysia) can suppress the growth of breast cancer cells. Although there is no reliable evidence demonstrating that this effect remains true in human clinical trials, it is reasonable to include honey as the sweetener of choice in patients with breast cancer.

Intravenous chemotherapy lines: When an intravenous line is inserted for the purpose of administering medication or chemotherapy, one of the concerns is infection at the entry point of the line. Studies have demonstrated that application of sterile medical grade honey (Surgihoney) directly at the site of the line can prevent or eradicate vascular line-site infections.

> *Concerning the generation of animals akin to them, as hornets and wasps, the facts in all cases are similar to a certain extent, but are devoid of the extraordinary features which characterize bees; this we should expect, for they have nothing divine about them as the bees have.*
>
> ~ Aristotle 384 BC - 322 BC

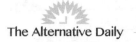

Part II Honey and Bee Questions and Answers

Question: *Can I give honey to my child?*

Despite all of the amazing benefits of honey, it should not be used on children under 1 year of age. This recommendation is based on the possibility of infants developing a rare but very serious condition called infantile botulism. The micro-organism that causes this potentially fatal condition has been found in small amounts in selected honey samples all over the world. A mature immune system is not vulnerable to this low level exposure, but the immature immune and gastro-intestinal systems of an infant make babies much more vulnerable. Infantile botulism is a real and serious disease that is associated with the consumption of honey by babies, and the recommendation to avoid honey and honey-flavored products until after age one is wise.

Question: *How much honey should I take daily?*

Unless you are using honey to treat a specific problem, most people can safely enjoy 2-3 teaspoons of honey per day. I add about 1 teaspoon to my coffee or tea.

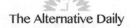

Question: Does cheap honey found in the grocery store do the same thing as raw, unpasteurized honey?

Absolutely not! The inexpensive honey that is found on store shelves is a far cry from raw, unfiltered, unpasteurized honey from a local beekeeper. Just like many highly processed food products, the contents of that cheap honey scarcely resembles honey fresh from the hive. Commercial honey products are often heated to high temperatures, filtered, and sometimes even adulterated with added color, flavor and even other sweeteners. This processing is used to remove tiny particles, including pollen grains, helps to keep the honey from crystallizing and maintains the color and clarity that consumers often prefer. I prefer and advise people to buy minimally processed local honey.

Question: If honey does not go bad, why does it have a "best before" date?

When it comes to expiration or "best before" dates, honey really is an exception. Honey that is properly stored in a sealed container is stable for decades (and even centuries). Over time, even properly stored honey may change color and flavor, but it does not "go bad" in a way that is dangerous. Always use a clean utensil to remove honey from the jar. If you're like me, there is never any concern about honey going bad, because I polish it off quick!

Question: Can I use honey if I have diabetes?

Although it may come as a surprise, newer research has suggested that in addition to all of the important nutritional do's and don'ts for diabetes, moderate amounts of honey can be used safely in diabetic patients. There do appear to be some individual differences in the way diabetics respond to the addition of

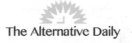

honey. So, in my diabetic patients who follow an otherwise healthy diet, I recommend that they consider adding up to one tablespoon of honey per day (usually in coffee or tea) and measure and track how their blood sugar responds.

Question: *Is it true that the government is using bees to sniff out bombs?*

It's true that bees and wasps have been studied for inclusion in the bomb squad. Although they are not widely or routinely used for this purpose, it is quite clear that bees and wasps are indeed capable of being trained to detect explosives.

Question: *Do bees poop in their honey?*

Honey is not made of bee poop. Although bees do indeed poop (just like everybody else), they generally do this away from the hive where the honey is produced. Bees eat the honey they make… would you poop in your kitchen? Hopefully not! And in case you were worried, honey is not made of bee vomit either.

Question: *Can I give honey to my pets?*

Yes! Integrative veterinarians use honey in pets for many of the same problems for which it is used for in humans. Allergies, respiratory problems and skin problems can all be good indications for honey in household pets. Honey should be avoided in baby dogs and cats under 6 months old. Beyond that, raw, local honey can be used externally on skin and internally at a dose of about ¼- ½ teaspoon per 20 pounds of body weight.

Question: *Will eating too much honey rot my teeth?*

There is some evidence that manuka honey may actually help prevent dental plaque and decay because of its antibacterial properties. This is an interesting finding indeed, but I would not start brushing your teeth or rinsing your mouth with honey just yet. Eating well and brushing and flossing your teeth are still the most important ways to take care of your teeth.

Question: *Can I be allergic to certain types of honey?*

Yes. People can indeed be allergic to honey, and ingestion of honey by these individuals can be dangerous. Studies have been performed in these individuals to identify what components of the honey may be inducing the allergic reaction. The results suggest that honey allergy can be caused by:

1. Components related to bee venom that "cross react" in people who are also allergic to bee stings.
2. Pollen grains in the honey that individuals are allergic to.
3. Components in the honey itself, independent of the bees that made it or the flower that it was made from.

Question: *If honey bees collect pollen from genetically modified plants and honey is made from it, will it hurt me?*

Unfortunately, the only way I can answer this question truthfully is to say… I don't know. It is very difficult (basically impossible) for beekeepers to prevent their bees from collecting pollen from fields growing GM crops. Therefore, the pollen from those crops can and does wind up in the honey. Pollen from GM crops has

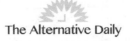

indeed been found in honey and this concerns me greatly. The health effects from consuming this GM pollen in honey are unknown. This is yet another reason to buy locally-produced honey rather than the large scale, commercially produced kind.

Question: How do I use honey as a sugar substitute in cooking or baking?

Honey is sweeter than sugar, so the general rule is to use about half as much honey as you would sugar (ie. If a recipe calls for 1 cup of sugar, use ½ cup of honey). Since honey is a liquid, you must also decrease the liquid content in the recipe if you substitute honey for sugar. For each cup of honey that is used in a recipe, reduce the other liquid in the recipe by ¼ cup. Also, when baking with honey, it is generally a good idea to reduce the temperature by about 25 degrees.

Question: My honey turned cloudy and thick...is it ok?

Yes. Your honey has crystallized, but it is perfectly fine. Crystallization is a natural process that results when the sugars in honey separate from the liquid portion. In some ways, crystallized honey is easier to use and less messy than the liquid. However, if you prefer liquid honey, try gently heating the honey in a warm water bath and stirring until the crystals dissolve.

Question: The honey I just bought looks and tastes different than the honey I'm used to.

Honey is a natural product and there are many factors that influence its aroma, flavor, color and clarity. Each honey is unique... enjoy the subtle differences from batch to batch.

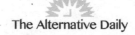

The True Liquid Gold

Honey is truly a gift that has earned its reputation as 'liquid gold." After reading this book, it should be evident that honey is not just a sweet and delicious treat - it is also a nutritionally dense food with amazing therapeutic value.

It should also be clear that bees work very, very hard all day long to collect enough pollen to make honey - they are, in many respects, working for us. We should have the utmost respect for these insects and the work that they do. This realization may cause you to become sensitive to the things that are threatening the health and vitality of our world's bees.

Enjoy honey and all it has to offer!

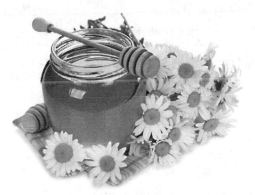

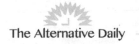

Sources:

1. http://www.benefits-of-honey.com/bee.html

2. http://www.ncbi.nlm.nih.gov/pubmed/11485891

3. http://www.americanjournalofsurgery.com/article/0002-9610(83)90204-0/pdf

4. http://www.ncbi.nlm.nih.gov/pubmed/17113690

5. http://www.ncbi.nlm.nih.gov/pubmed/15130571

6. http://www.ncbi.nlm.nih.gov/pubmed/15117561

7. http://ijl.sagepub.com/content/5/1/40.abstract

8. http://www.ncbi.nlm.nih.gov/pubmed/12171686

9. http://www.ncbi.nlm.nih.gov/pubmed/15278008

10. http://onlinelibrary.wiley.com/store/10.1111/fct.12078/asset/fct12078.pdf?v=1&t=i2no3990&s=54beefb13c3e42087ec8929383a8678e9d7bcb14

11. http://onlinelibrary.wiley.com/doi/10.1111/j.1479-828X.1992.tb02861.x/abstract;jsessionid=059D94F9F53A4EBC34A97413076DCE60.d04t02

12. http://www.ncbi.nlm.nih.gov/pmc/articles/PMC3758027

13. http://som.adzu.edu.ph/research/pdf/2008-05-19-160455aujero,a..pdf

14. http://www.ncbi.nlm.nih.gov/pubmed/17031045

15. http://www.medicinenet.com/script/main/art.asp?articlekey=50602

16. http://www.health24.com/Natural/Natural-living/The-health-benefits-of-honey-20130523

17. http://www.webmd.com/diet/features/medicinal-uses-of-honey

18. http://www.sciencedaily.com/releases/2014/03/140316132801.htm

19. http://www.revbiomed.uady.mx/pdf/rb96716.pdf

20. http://www.ncbi.nlm.nih.gov/pubmed/17413836

21. http://www.ncbi.nlm.nih.gov/pmc/articles/PMC1292197

22. http://www.sciencedirect.com/science/article/pii/S0378874104002995

23. http://www.biomedcentral.com/1472-6882/9/34/

24. http://researchcommons.waikato.ac.nz/handle/10289/2059

25. http://journals.lww.com/jwocnonline/Abstract/2002/11000/Honey__A_Potent_Agent_for_Wound_Healing_.8.aspx

The Alternative Daily

26. http://rcnpublishing.com/doi/abs/10.7748/ns2000.11.15.11.63.c2952

27. http://www.hindawi.com/journals/ecam/2009/620857/abs

28. http://www.tandfonline.com/doi/abs/10.1080/02791072.1981.10471447?journalCode=ujpd20

29. http://researchcommons.waikato.ac.nz/handle/10289/2140

30. http://link.springer.com/article/10.1007/s10096-009-0763-z

31. http://www.sciencedirect.com/science/article/pii/S2221169111600166

32. http://medscimonit.com/abstract/index/idArt/11736

33. http://link.springer.com/article/10.1007/s12349-009-0051-6#page-1

34. http://online.liebertpub.com/doi/abs/10.1089/109629603766957022

35. http://researchcommons.waikato.ac.nz/handle/10289/2060

36. http://www.ncbi.nlm.nih.gov/pubmed/18666717

37. http://www.karger.com/Article/FullText/319821#tab4

38. http://www.ncbi.nlm.nih.gov/pubmed/15117561

39. http://www.ncbi.nlm.nih.gov/pubmed/12617614

40. http://onlinelibrary.wiley.com/doi/10.1111/j.1750-3841.2008.00966.x/full

41. http://www.ncbi.nlm.nih.gov/pmc/articles/PMC3821146/

42. http://link.springer.com/chapter/10.1007/978-1-4757-9371-0_3#page-1

43. http://www.cabdirect.org/abstracts/19970200985.html;jsessionid=B685908F325B3B980045FEAF0651309F

44. http://cat.inist.fr/?aModele=afficheN&cpsidt=14537419

45. http://www.ncbi.nlm.nih.gov/pmc/articles/PMC3263128/#!po=2.17391

46. http://www.jdmdonline.com/content/13/1/23

47. http://www.ncbi.nlm.nih.gov/pubmed/22114423

48. http://www.ncbi.nlm.nih.gov/pubmed/15125017

REVERSE AGING with Liquid Gold
DIY: Honey for Beauty

Your skin is your body's largest organ. Whatever you're putting on (or in) your body, including conditioner, deodorant, toothpaste and lotion, is being absorbed and either encouraging good health or wreaking havoc on your system.

Do you know what's in your skin care products? Many products we use contain harsh chemicals, parabens (which have been linked to cancer) and other artificial ingredients.

Want to know a few skin care ingredients that may be causing problems for your health?

1. **Parabens.** Ingredients like methylparaben and butylparaben are common in a lot of beauty products. They have been found in breast cancer tumors and have been linked to serious long-term diseases. They're also considered endocrine disrupters and can cause reproductive problems.

Avoid products with parabens at all costs.

2. **Fragrance.** Unless you're using a product that's scented with essential oils, most companies use chemicals to artificially create a scent. Besides creating an allergy issue, chemical-laden fragrances can lead to hormone disruption. To be safe, choose products made with essential oils or natural scents.

3. **Preservatives.** To extend the life of products (so they don't spoil), companies use preservatives such as methylisothiazolinone and methylchloroisothiazolinone, which may have neurotoxic properties.

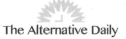

The Alternative Daily

Look at the labels of the products you're using and make sure they're not laden with preservatives.

Honey - Nature's Answer

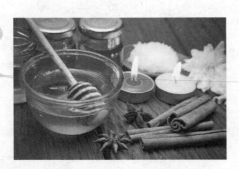

Not only are honey's therapeutic health properties well known, it is also known that honey has the ability to help you look your best. Cleopatra herself used honey as an integral part of her beauty routine.

Honey is a natural humectant, meaning it not only draws moisture from the air and keeps skin hydrated, it is also loaded with enzymes and anti-oxidants, as well as anti-inflammatory and nourishing properties that clean and feed the skin. All of this without the worry of dangerous chemicals!

Honey Beauty Recipes

Here are a few of our favorite honey beauty recipes to keep you glowing and looking great.

Makeup Remover

Ingredients:

- Honey
- Organic coconut oil

Instructions:

1. Mix enough honey and coconut oil together to form a spreadable mixture.

2. Apply to face (do not get in eyes), then rinse with warm water.

3. Pat dry.

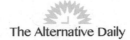
The Alternative Daily

Honey Sunburn Treatment
◇◇◇◇◇◇◇◇◇◇◇◇◇

Ingredients:

- 1 part raw honey
- 2 parts pure aloe vera

Instructions:

Mix the ingredients together and apply to sore skin.

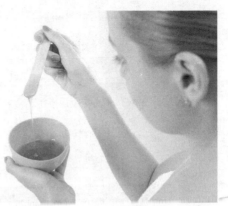

Coconut Honey Hair Mask
◇◇◇◇◇◇◇◇◇◇◇◇

Ingredients:

- 2 tablespoons coconut oil
- 2 tablespoons honey

Instructions:

1. Heat the honey and coconut oil in a small saucepan until well combined and warm.

2. Apply hair mask to damp hair.

3. Run your fingers or a wide tooth comb through your hair to distribute the mask evenly.

4. Wrap your hair into a bun and allow the mask to sit for 30-40 minutes.

5. Rinse clean with warm water.

Dark Circle Remover
◇◇◇◇◇◇◇◇◇◇◇

Ingredients:

- 1 teaspoon honey
- 1 teaspoon sweet almond oil

Instructions:

1. Mix ingredients together and apply under eyes.

2. Allow mixture to sit for 20 minutes, then rinse off with warm water and pat dry.

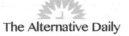

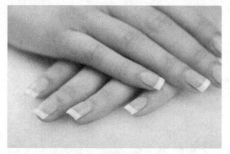

Cuticle Moisturizer

Ingredients:

- 1 teaspoon honey
- 1 teaspoon apple cider vinegar
- 1 teaspoon coconut oil

Instructions;

1. Mix all ingredients together.
2. Apply to cuticles and let set for 10 minutes.
3. Rinse off with warm water
4. Pat dry.

Nail Strengthening Treatment

Ingredients:

- 1 tablespoon honey
- 1/4 cup apple cider vinegar

Instructions:

1. Mix ingredients together in a shallow dish.
2. Soak nails in mixture for 10 minutes.
3. Rinse clean.

Peppermint Honey Foot Scrub

Ingredients:

- 1/4 cup brown sugar
- 2 tablespoons coconut oil
- 3 tablespoons honey
- 3 drop peppermint essential oil

Instructions:

1. Mix all ingredients together well.
2. Apply to feet using a circular scrubbing motion.
3. Rinse clean with warm water. Towel dry.

The Alternative Daily

Honey Body Lotion

◇◇◇◇◇◇◇◇◇◇◇

Ingredients:

- 1 tablespoon honey
- 1/2 cup grated beeswax
- 200 ml almond oil
- 1/2 cup rosewater

Instructions:

1. Heat honey, beeswax and almond oil together in a small saucepan.

2. Once everything is mixed together well and melted, remove from heat.

3. Allow to cool slightly.

4. Add rosewater to the lotion one drop at a time, whisking while adding.

5. Pour cream into a jar.

6. Allow to cool before closing jar.

Citrus Honey Face Mask

◇◇◇◇◇◇◇◇◇◇◇◇◇

Ingredients:

- Boiling water
- 1/2 lemon
- 1 tablespoon honey

Instructions:

1. Pour boiling water in a bowl and stand over the steam. This will open your pores and allow them to soak in the benefits of the mask.

2. Mix the lemon and honey together and apply as a mask to your face, avoiding the eye area.

3. Let the mask sit for 15 minutes.

4. Rinse clean with warm water.

5. Splash cold water on your face to close your pores.

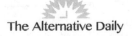

The Alternative Daily

Honey Lavender Chap Stick

Ingredients:

- 2 tablespoons coconut oil
- 1 tablespoon shea butter
- 1/2 teaspoon honey
- 1 tablespoon sweet almond oil
- 2 tablespoons beeswax
- 15 drops lavender essential oil
- 5 drops frankincense essential oil
- 12 empty lip balm tubes and a rubber band.

Instructions:

1. Remove the caps from the lip balm tubes and bundle them together with a rubber band.

2. Melt the coconut oil, shea butter, honey, beeswax and essential oils together in a double boiler.

3. Remove from heat and stir in almond oil.

4. Quickly pour mixture into lip balm tubes before the wax sets.

5. Put the lids on the containers and allow to harden.

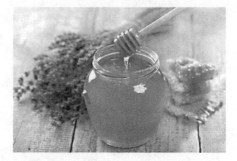

Honey Hair Deep Conditioner

Ingredients:

- 1 tablespoon honey
- 1 tablespoon olive oil

Instructions:

1. Mix honey and olive oil together in a small sauce pot.

2. Heat mixture just until warm.

3. Apply mixture to wet hair and comb through evenly.

4. Wrap hair in a warm towel and let the conditioner soak in for 20-30 minutes.

5. Rinse out and shampoo as normal.

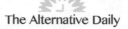

The Alternative Daily

Honey Bath Soak

Ingredients:

- 1/2 cup honey
- 2 cups organic milk
- 8 drops eucalyptus essential oil

Instructions:

Add all ingredients to running water in a hot bath.

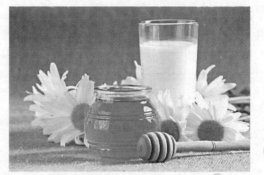

Coconut Honey Bath Soak

Ingredients:

- 2 cups coconut milk
- 4 tablespoons honey
- 10 drops of your favorite essential oil

Instructions:

1. Mix all ingredients together in a bowl.
2. Once well combined, pour into a warm bath.
3. Stir the water around with your hand before soaking.

Brown Sugar Honey Face Scrub

Ingredients:

- 1/4 cup raw honey
- 1/4 cup brown sugar

Instructions:

1. Place honey and sugar in a small jar with a lid.
2. Mix together well.
3. Apply to wet face in a circular scrubbing motion.
4. Rinse clean with cool water.

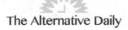

Citrus Honey Foot Soak

Ingredients:

- 1/2 cup honey
- 1/2 cup apple cider vinegar
- 1/2 lemon, sliced
- Hot water

Instructions:

1. Place honey, vinegar and lemon slices in a large bowl.

2. Add hot water over the previous ingredients.

3. Soak feet for 15-20 minutes, then towel dry.

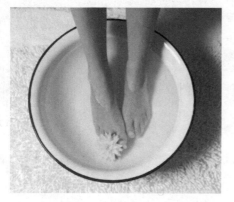

Honey Sugar Body Scrub

Ingredients:

- 1/4 cup honey
- 2 tablespoons coconut oil
- 1/2 cup brown sugar
- A few drops of essential oils (your choice)

Instructions:

1. Melt honey and coconut oil on the stove.

2. Add brown sugar and essential oils to mixture.

3. Stir to combine, then scrub all over damp skin in a gentle circular motion.

4. Rinse clean with warm water.

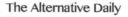

The Alternative Daily

Honey and Vinegar Fall Hair Treatment

Ingredients:

- 10 tablespoons apple cider vinegar
- 1/4 of honey

Instructions:

1. Mix honey and vinegar together.

2. Apply mixture to hair and massage in evenly.

3. Allow mixture to sit for 20 minutes, then wash clean.

Honey Olive Oil Lip Balm

Ingredients:

- 1 tablespoon honey, melted
- 1 tablespoon olive oil

Instructions:

1. Mix ingredients together and pour into a small container.

2. Allow lip balm to harden. Apply to lips as needed.

Milk and Honey Face Wash

Ingredients:

- 1/4 cup milk or cream
- 1 tablespoon honey

Instructions:

1. Mix honey and milk or cream together in a small dish.

2. Apply mixture to damp face.

3. Rinse clean with warm water to reveal glowing skin.

Bad Breath Treatment

Ingredients:

- 1/4 cup water
- 1 teaspoon honey
- 1 teaspoon lemon juice

Instructions:

1. Mix together all ingredients.

2. Gargle with mixture for 3 minutes. Rinse mouth clean.

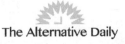

The Alternative Daily

Honey Baking Soda Scar Treatment

Ingredients:

- 1 tablespoon baking soda
- 1 tablespoon honey

Instructions:

1. Mix honey and baking soda together to create a paste.
2. Apply paste to scars.
3. Allow the paste to sit for 30 minutes, then rinse clean.

Honey Almond Exfoliator

Ingredients:

- 1/4 cup ground almonds
- 1/4 cup honey

Instructions:

1. Mix honey and almonds together.
2. Rub mixture in a circular motion onto damp skin.
3. Rinse clean.

Natural Hair Remover

Ingredients:

- 1 tablespoon honey
- 1 tablespoon lemon juice
- 3 tablespoons brown sugar

Instructions:

1. Combine all ingredients in a microwave safe bowl. Warm slightly in the microwave.
2. Allow mixture to cool and apply to facial hair using a popsicle stick.
3. Place a small piece of muslin cloth over the area and rub slightly.
4. Remove with a quick pull in the opposite direction of hair growth.

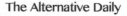

The Alternative Daily

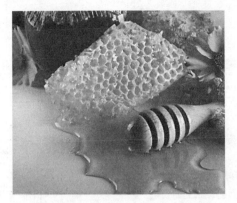

Skin Tightening Treatment

◇◇◇◇◇◇◇◇◇◇◇◇◇◇◇◇

Ingredients:

- 1 tablespoon honey
- White of 1 egg

Instructions:

1. Mix honey and egg white together to make a paste.

2. Apply to face.

3. Rinse clean after 15-20 minutes.

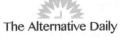

25 Healing Recipes
Honey in the Kitchen

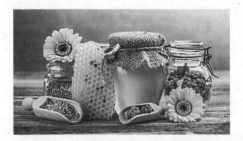

Incorporating honey into your diet is easy and delicious. Be sure that you use local, organic honey (and other ingredients) whenever possible.

Strawberry Honey Smoothie

Ingredients:

- 1 cup strawberries
- 1 tablespoon honey
- 1 teaspoon vanilla
- 1 cup milk
- 1 frozen banana

Instructions:

Blend all ingredients in a blender until well combined. Pour into a glass and enjoy.

Greek Honey Parfait

Ingredients:

- 2 cups Greek yogurt
- 2 tablespoons honey
- 1 cup fresh fruit

Instructions:

1. Place a few tablespoons of yogurt in the bottom of two glasses.

2. Top the yogurt with a drizzle of honey and a bit of fruit.

3. Continue until the glasses are full.

4. Serve while fresh.

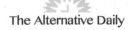

Honey Lemon Tea

Ingredients:

- 1 tablespoon freshly squeezed lemon juice
- 2 tablespoons honey
- 1 cup boiling water

Instructions:

1. Squeeze the lemon juice into a mug.
2. Add the honey and stir.
3. Pour boiling water over the honey and lemon. Stir, and enjoy while warm.

Cinnamon Spiced Honey Butter

Ingredients:

- 1/4 pound unsalted butter
- 4 tablespoons honey
- 1/2 teaspoon cinnamon
- 1/4 teaspoon salt

Instructions:

1. Using a mixer with a paddle attachment, mix all ingredients together.
2. Serve honey butter at room temperature.

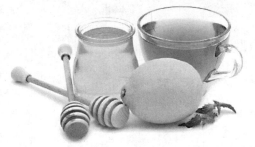

The Alternative Daily

Honey Almond Smoothie

◇◇◇◇◇◇◇◇◇◇◇◇◇

Ingredients:

- 1 1/2 cups almond milk
- 1/4 cup almond butter
- 2 tablespoons honey
- 1 tablespoon cinnamon
- 1 frozen banana

Instructions:

Place all ingredients in a blender. Mix on high until smooth.

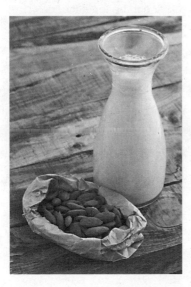

Easy Honey Fruit Dip

◇◇◇◇◇◇◇◇◇◇◇◇◇

Ingredients:

- 1 cup Greek yogurt
- 1/2 teaspoon cinnamon
- 1 teaspoon vanilla
- 4 tablespoons honey

Instructions:

1. Combine all ingredients in a bowl.
2. Chill before serving.

Mint-Infused Honey

◇◇◇◇◇◇◇◇◇◇◇◇◇

Ingredients:

- 2 cups honey
- 1/2 cup dry mint leaves

Instructions:

1. Place honey and mint in a cast iron pot.
2. Simmer on low heat until it almost reaches a boil.
3. Once cool, pour honey into a jar through a cheesecloth to strain out the mint leaves. Store in a cool, dark place.

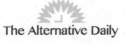

The Alternative Daily

Honey Carrot Soup

Ingredients:

- 2 cups carrots
- 4 cups vegetable broth
- 1/4 cup honey
- 3 cloves garlic, crushed
- Salt and pepper to taste
- 1 cup heavy cream
- Chopped parsley for garnish

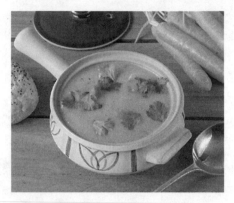

Instructions:

1. Peel and slice carrots.
2. Put carrots, broth, honey, garlic and salt and pepper in a sauce pan.
3. Bring soup to a boil, then simmer for 30 minutes.
4. Puree soup in a blender, then pour back into pot.
5. Stir in cream and serve topped with parsley.

Fruit and Nut Honey Butter

Ingredients:

- 1/2 cup butter, softened
- 1/4 cup walnuts
- 1/4 cup dried fruit

Instructions:

1. Mix together all ingredients with a whisk.
2. Refrigerate until solid.
3. Spread on gluten-free crackers or bread.

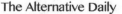

The Alternative Daily

Almond Honey Cake

◇◇◇◇◇◇◇◇◇◇

Ingredients:

- 4 cups almond flour
- 2 teaspoon baking powder
- 1 teaspoon baking soda
- 1 teaspoon cardamom
- 1 teaspoon ground ginger
- 1 teaspoon sea salt
- 3 eggs, beaten
- 1/3 cup of honey
- 1/4 cup coconut oil
- 6 ounces of raspberries
- Pistachios for garnish

Instructions:

1. Preheat oven to 350 degrees Fahrenheit. Grease two 9 inch pans with butter and dust with almond flour.

2. Whisk together dry ingredients.

3. Combine wet ingredients in a separate bowl. Fold in raspberries. Mix in the dry ingredients and put batter into pans.

4. Bake for 45 minutes or until a toothpick comes out clean.

5. Sprinkle top of cake with pistachios and serve.

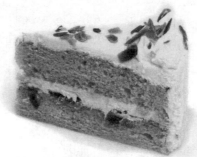

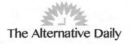

The Alternative Daily

Honey Cookies

◇◇◇◇◇◇◇◇

Ingredients:

- 1 cup honey
- ⅓ cup coconut oil
- 2 eggs
- 1 cup almond milk
- 3 1/2 cups gluten-free oat flour
- 1/2 cup brown rice flour
- 2 teaspoons baking powder
- 1/2 teaspoon baking soda
- 1 teaspoon cinnamon
- 1/2 teaspoon nutmeg

Instructions:

1. Preheat oven to 375 degrees Fahrenheit.

2. Combine the oil and honey together. Stir eggs and milk into the mixture.

3. Sift dry ingredients together, then combine with honey mixture.

4. Place dough by teaspoons on greased baking sheet and bake for 12 minutes or until lightly brown.

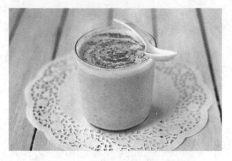

Honey and Peanut Butter Milkshake

◇◇◇◇◇◇◇◇◇◇◇◇◇◇◇◇

Ingredients:

- 1/2 cup milk
- 1 tablespoon peanut butter
- 1 tablespoon ground flax seed
- 2 teaspoons honey
- 1/2 teaspoon vanilla extract
- 1/2 teaspoon apple cider vinegar
- 1/4 teaspoon cinnamon
- 1 pinch sea salt
- 1 frozen banana
- 1 teaspoon raw cacao nibs for garnish.

Instructions:

Blend until smooth. Pour into a glass and top with cacao nibs.

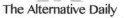

The Alternative Daily

Honey Almond Bars

◇◇◇◇◇◇◇◇◇◇

Ingredients:

- 1 cup rolled oats
- 1/4 cup slivered almonds
- 1/4 cup sunflower seeds
- 1 tablespoon flax seeds
- 1 tablespoon sesame seeds
- 1 cup gluten-free puff cereal
- 1/3 cup currants
- 1/3 cup dried apricots
- 1/3 cup raisins
- 1/4 cup almond butter
- 1/4 cup coconut sugar
- 1/4 cup honey
- 1/2 teaspoon vanilla extract
- Pinch of salt

Instructions:

1. Preheat oven to 350 degrees Fahrenheit.

2. Spread oats, almonds, flax and sesame seeds on a lightly greased baking sheet.

3. Bake until toasted, or about 10 minutes. Shake frequently

4. Transfer oats, nuts, and seeds to a bowl and add cereal and fruit. Shake to mix.

5. Combine the remaining ingredients in a saucepan and heat until bubbly.

6. Pour heated liquid over dry ingredients in a bowl and combine well.

7. Transfer mixture to the greased pan. Coat your hands in coconut oil and press mixture down to form to the pan.

8. Refrigerate for 30 minutes or until hard. Cut into bars and enjoy.

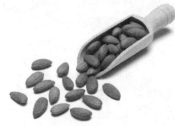

Lavender Honey Ice Cream

◇◇◇◇◇◇◇◇◇◇◇◇◇◇◇

Ingredients:

- 2 cups heavy cream
- 1 cup half and half
- 2/3 cup honey
- 2 tablespoons dried lavender flowers
- 2 eggs
- 1/8 teaspoon salt

Instructions:

1. Bring cream, half and half, honey and lavender to a boil over medium heat. Stir frequently.

2. Remove from heat and let steep, covered, for 30 minutes, then strain through a sieve to remove the lavender flowers.

3. In a large bowl, whisk the salt and eggs together, then slowly add the cream mixture.

4. Cook over low heat, stirring constantly with a wooden spoon until thickened. Allow to cool.

5. Chill in the fridge for 3 hours, then freeze in an ice cream maker when ready to serve.

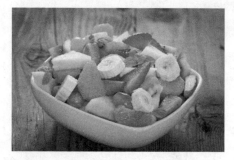

Honey Fruit Salad

◇◇◇◇◇◇◇◇◇◇

Ingredients:

- 1 orange, sliced
- 1 cup of pineapple, cubed
- 1 cup grapes
- 1 cup strawberries, chopped
- 1 banana, sliced
- 4 tablespoons honey
- 2 tablespoons lime juice
- 1 teaspoon vanilla extract
- 1/4 teaspoon poppy seeds
- 2 teaspoons lime zest

Instructions:

Place all ingredients into a bowl. Toss to combine. Chill before serving.

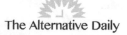

Garlic Honey Chicken

◇◇◇◇◇◇◇◇◇◇◇◇

Ingredients

- 1 cup coconut flour
- 1 1/2 teaspoons baking powder
- 1/2 teaspoon sea salt
- 3/4 cup water
- 1/3 cup sesame seeds
- Coconut oil for frying
- 1 1/2 pounds boneless, skinless, free-range chicken breasts, cubed
- 1/2 cup honey
- 2 garlic cloves, minced
- 1/4 teaspoon liquid aminos

Instructions:

1. Mix batter for chicken by combining flour, baking soda, salt, and water.

2. Toast the sesame seeds in a deep skillet until brown.

3. Reduce heat and add oil to the skillet so the bottom is covered. Heat until oil is hot.

4. Dip both sides of chicken in batter, then cook in skillet.

5. Mix honey, garlic and liquid aminos in a bowl. Pour over cooked chicken. Best if served right away.

Honey Salad Dressing

◇◇◇◇◇◇◇◇◇◇◇◇

Ingredients:

- 1/3 cup white balsamic vinegar
- 2 tablespoons honey
- 1 tablespoon dijon mustard
- 1/2 teaspoon salt
- 1/2 teaspoon pepper
- 2/3 cup olive oil

Instructions:

Whisk all ingredients together. Drizzle over your favorite salad.

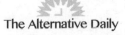

The Alternative Daily

Honey Glazed Carrots

◇◇◇◇◇◇◇◇◇◇◇◇

Ingredients:

- 1 pound baby carrots
- 2 tablespoons butter
- 2 tablespoons honey
- 2 teaspoons apple cider vinegar
- Salt and pepper to taste

Instructions:

1. Steam carrots above an inch of water until tender.

2. Melt butter in a saucepan and mix in vinegar and honey.

3. Saute the tender carrots in the honey mixture until well-coated.

4. Serve while warm.

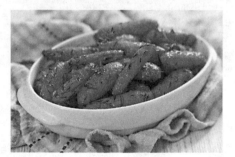

Chilled Honey Lemon Juice

◇◇◇◇◇◇◇◇◇◇◇◇◇

Ingredients:

- 2 tablespoons fresh lemon juice
- 2 tablespoons honey
- 8 cups cold water
- A pinch of sea salt
- A pinch of black pepper

Instructions:

1. Mix all ingredients together in a pitcher.

2. Pour into chilled glasses and enjoy

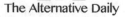

The Alternative Daily

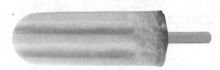

Frozen Honey Fruit Bars

Ingredients:

- 1 kiwi, sliced
- 10 strawberries, chopped
- Pulp of 1 orange
- 10 grapes, sliced
- 3 tablespoons honey
- 1/2 cup green tea

Instructions:

1. Arrange the slices of fruit along the sides of 4 popsicle molds.

2. Mix green tea and honey. Pour mixture into popsicle molds.

3. Freeze for 8 hours or until solid.

Tropical Honey Popsicles

Ingredients:

- 4 cups coconut milk
- 1 4-inch piece of ginger, grated finley
- 1 cup honey

Instructions:

1. Place milk, ginger and honey in a heavy-bottomed sauce pan.

2. Bring mixture to a boil over medium heat.

3. Cook at a simmer until honey is dissolved.

4. Reduce heat and cook on low for 10 additional minutes.

5. Strain the mixture through a fine mesh sieve. Allow it to cool to room temperature.

6. Pour mixture into popsicle molds. Add a popsicle stick to each mold, cover, and freeze until solid.

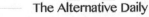

Cinnamon Honey Sweet Potatoes

Ingredients:

- 4 sweet potatoes, peeled and cubed
- 1/4 cup olive oil
- 1/4 cup honey
- 2 teaspoons cinnamon
- Salt and pepper to taste

Instructions:

1. Preheat oven to 375 Fahrenheit.
2. Lay the cubed potatoes in a single layer on a roasting tray.
3. Drizzle with the oil and honey. Sprinkle on cinnamon, salt and pepper.
4. Roast for 25 minutes or until tender.

Cinnamon Honey Oatmeal

Ingredients:

- 4 cups cooked steel-cut oats
- 2 cups half and half
- 1/4 cup honey
- 1 tablespoon cinnamon

Instructions:

1. Mix warm cooked oats with half and half.
2. Serve oatmeal into bowls.
3. Drizzle with honey and cinnamon.

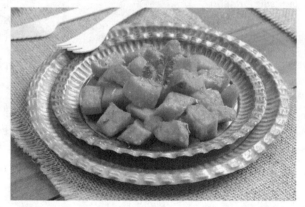

The Alternative Daily

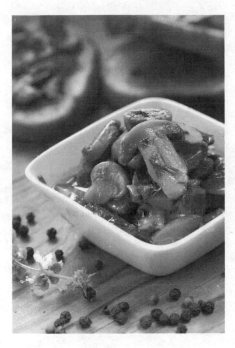

Honey Mushrooms

◇◇◇◇◇◇◇◇◇◇

Ingredients:

- 5 leaves of lettuce
- 1 cup chopped mushrooms
- Salt and pepper to taste
- 4 cloves garlic, chopped
- 2 tablespoons coconut oil
- 3 tablespoons balsamic vinegar
- 1 tablespoon honey

Instructions:

1. Heat coconut oil in skillet until melted. Add garlic and cook until slightly brown.

2. Add mushrooms and cook until soft.

3. Add salt and pepper as desired.

4. Remove from heat. Add lettuce, honey and vinegar to mixture. Toss in a large bowl and serve.

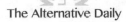

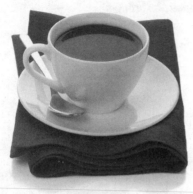

Honey Hot Cocoa

◇◇◇◇◇◇◇◇◇◇

Ingredients:

- 2 tablespoons honey
- 2 tablespoons raw cocoa powder
- Pinch of sea salt
- 1 cup milk

Instructions:

1. Whisk all ingredients together in a saucepan.

2. Cook over medium heat until simmering.

3. Serve while warm.

The Alternative Daily

*The Natural Remedies
That May Halt, Reverse and
Even Cure Many Diseases*

Natural
Cures

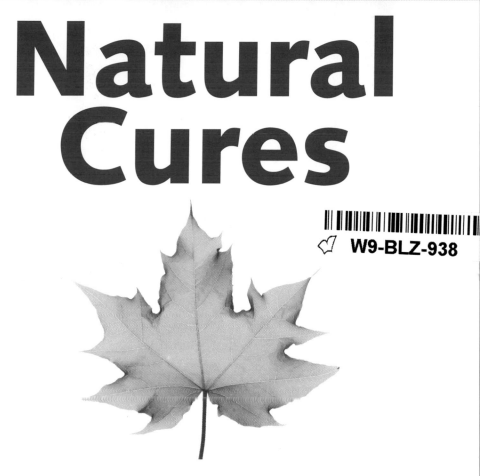

W9-BLZ-938

FROM A REAL MEDICAL DOCTOR

Allen S. Josephs, M.D.

*A Common Sense
Action Guide for Optimal
Health & Longevity*

Manufactured in the United States of America
First Edition

Table of Contents

❦ Introduction

On January 10, 1776, a man by the name of Thomas Paine changed the world. *Common Sense*, his 46-page pamphlet, burned through the consciousness of Americans and fueled their desire to throw off their oppressive British rule, leading to the American Revolution and an entirely new political experiment called democracy. Prior to Paine's *Common Sense*, most citizens of the 13 colonies wanted to appease King George and their British government and avoid a revolution at all costs.

Today, 230 years later, this 46-page book in honor of Thomas Paine is, likewise, a call for revolution, not against our democracy, but rather against the current health care system that is putting our great country, U.S. companies and our fellow citizens into bankruptcy.

Health care costs continue to skyrocket out of control and dramatically outpace overall growth in this country. We are now spending a staggering $1.7 trillion a year, 14 percent of our gross domestic product (GDP) on health care. This is more than 300 percent of the amount most countries spend on health care.

I grew up hearing, "As General Motors (GM) goes, so goes the country." GM, as you are probably aware, is in poor financial condition. It has lost its competitive edge and may face bankruptcy. GM's financial problems are due, in part, to the tremendous cost of the health care program the company provides for its employees. In fact, shockingly, GM spends more on health care costs than on steel for its cars!

I could understand if these tremendous costs provided us with the best health care and disease-free life in the world. Sadly, this is not the case. In a 2001 Canadian study of eight developed nations, the United States was placed number four in terms of quality medical care, after Singapore, Britain and Canada, all of which spend considerably less per capita than we do. In another study based on infant mortality, our status is even worse, with the U.S. ranking near the bottom of the list at number 28. That means 27 other countries rank higher, and spend far less than we do.

The average American family spends between $10,000 and $12,000 a year for health insurance and health care costs. If that family was able to invest this money in a typical mutual fund instead, within 20 to 25 years there would be $1 million in the bank for that family's pleasure, security and retirement. We've all heard the tragic stories of families forced into bankruptcy by health care costs, losing their homes, and their dignity.

Is this fair? Of course not!

Can we change this broken down system? Yes!

We can change it with knowledge and action.

Unfortunately, we Americans have been lulled into a false sense of security about our health care system. Drug companies run expensive ads making us believe they have cures for our diseases. Hospitals run ads making us think they can cure atherosclerotic heart disease and other degenerative disorders.

Even more disturbing is the avalanche of so-called "information" about the best ways to create our own health. Much of it is misleading, some of it is downright wrong. Worst of all, some is even fraudulent. No wonder we're confused!

Partly as a result of all of this misinformation, we abuse our bodies by not exercising, taking no vitamins or ineffective ones, eating toxic foods, smoking and drinking excessively.

Then when we get sick, we believe the doctors and drug companies will provide a magical cure in the form of a pill or surgery. I'll let you in on a big secret: That "magical cure" does not exist for most people and for most diseases.

When I started medical school more than 30 years ago, I believed that doctors, drug companies and hospitals had all the answers. Over these last couple of decades, I learned that, for the most part, doctors are only able to treat symptoms. Treating those symptoms comes at great cost, financially, physically and emotionally. The treatment often causes side effects, the disease eventually progresses and may cause us to become disabled or even to die.

Medical science can cure almost nothing beyond bacterial infections if the correct antibiotic is chosen or patch you up if you're in an accident.

For example, just look at the way we treat cancer in the year 2006: We cut it out, burn it out or poison it, just like we did 40 years ago. All of these therapies will further impair or even destroy immune function—one of the main reasons why the cancer became a problem in the first place. This kind of treatment is completely illogical. Although some cancers can be "cured" with these various therapies if they're caught early, many times the treatment can have devastating effects, even worse than the cancer itself.

Doctors mean well, but most physicians have been taught to treat illnesses with drugs and surgery. True, we were also taught in medical school how cells function and the importance of proper nutrients like essential fatty acids, magnesium, B vitamins, zinc, carnitine and CoQ10 to keep those cells healthy. Yet, somewhere along the line, we doctors lost sight of this information, ignoring these safe, effective and inexpensive natural remedies.

Our soaring health problems are destroying not only our bodies but the health of our families and our country's financial health. We are truly bankrupting our children's, grandchildren's and great-grandchildren's health and wealth.

Now is the time for each and every one of us to take responsibility for our health and our families' health. It's time to declare a revolution against our current unhealthy lifestyles and the over consumption of drugs, surgery and hospitalization in favor of natural health and cures. Thomas Paine's wisdom rings as true today as he said over 200 years ago, "A long habit of not thinking a thing wrong gives it a superficial appearance of being right." This is truly the state of most people's and doctors' belief system with our current failed health care system.

Join me on this journey. The tools I offer you in this book will help you choose natural cures to regain and maintain optimal health and longevity while reducing or eliminating dangerous drugs, invasive procedures and toxic foods. As the most honorable and brilliant Thomas Paine said, "Virtues are acquired through endeavor, which rests wholly upon yourself."

Choose natural health and enjoy a long, healthy and happy life you can easily create for yourself and for your family. By doing this, one family at a time, we will solve our health care crisis.

Allen S. Josephs, M.D.
January 10, 2006

Chapter 1
*Changes to save your life
and the lives of future generations*

If you're as old as I am, you'll remember the comic strip character, a swamp possum named Pogo. One of Pogo's most famous pronouncements was, "I've met the enemy and he is us."

Pogo's wisdom has never been more relevant than it is today.

We have, in so many ways, become our own worst enemy.

This is your call to action. Now is the time to take responsibility for your own health. No one else can do this for you.

It would be easy to blame our problems on hospitals, insurance companies, drug companies and doctors. Certainly they bear a great deal of responsibility for today's medical and financial disasters. Yet I suggest to you now that the major share of the responsibility lands squarely on your shoulders and the shoulders of every single American citizen.

Your body cannot be replaced. Doctors can only go so far to repair it when you abuse it. So why not value yourself, feed yourself only the highest quality, freshest and healthiest foods, delight in your body's ability to move with ease and wake up each morning eager to greet another day of vibrant life? You deserve it!

I am going to provide you a quick and concise action plan to jumpstart you on the path of excellent health and long life. If you're groaning about draconian diets and four-hour daily workouts, let me assure you that this is a simple and easy plan. It's packed with small changes that can make big differences in your health and even prevent, reverse and cure many common chronic diseases of aging, like diabetes, heart disease and cancer.

You can take baby steps with this plan or you can take giant leaps. It's your choice. But whatever steps you choose to take, you will be making important changes in your health and your life expectancy.

Exactly 230 years ago, Thomas Paine wrote in *Common Sense*, "We have it in our power to begin the world over again."

We, the American people and the health care system we have created, cannot be fixed by maintaining the status quo or by just shifting who pays for health care. Ultimately you will pay for your health care via taxes, less pay, lost jobs, higher insurance costs and perhaps with your life, since it is your health that is at stake.

The starting point
So where do we start?

FIRST: by taking a high quality multivitamin/mineral/antioxidant. Shockingly 50 percent of people fail to take any supplement. Just as bad is the fact less than 90 percent of those that do, take a low quality once a day that is grossly inadequate to provide any form of natural therapy or prevention for most common diseases.

SECOND: by controlling our weight. An appalling 64 percent of us are overweight and 30 percent of us are obese. The average American gets less than two servings of fruits and vegetables every day despite extensive research that proves that the simple act of eating at least five servings of fruits and vegetables a day is the single most beneficial thing you can do for your health and long life.

Not only are we eating junk, but we are feeding it to our children. A shocking 15 percent of our teenagers are overweight. The United States has the dubious honor of having the greatest percentage of overweight adolescents in the Western world. By feeding our children junk food, we are condemning them to a lifetime of weight-related health problems that surely will shorten their lives.

THIRD: by quitting smoking once and for all. I find it appalling that 23 percent of Americans still smoke. We know, without a doubt, that smoking causes a host of deadly health problems from numerous types of cancers to heart disease, stroke and the destruction of brain cells.

FOURTH: by cutting back on our drinking. Excessive alcohol consumption causes more than 100,000 deaths a year, ranging from drunk driving to cirrhosis of the liver, cancer and heart disease. While a 5-ounce glass or two of red wine a day is actually quite good for you, the line is very fine. Cross that line, and you're inviting serious troubles. What's more, hard liquor is highly toxic and increases mortality rates.

FIFTH: by exercising optimally. We have become a society of couch potatoes. Fewer than half of us get the daily recommended amount of daily exercise. Many of us are overweight because our over-stressed, over-fed lifestyles leave us with little time or energy for exercise.

FINALLY: by managing our stress. We are a stressed-out society. Nearly 75 percent of all visits to primary care physicians are stress-related, the American Psychological Association reports.

This puts an unbelievable burden on our staggering health care system and on our physical and emotional well-being.

I'm not judging you. I'm here to help you. Together, we can fix our bodies, minds, and yes, our spirits. The method does not have to be burdensome. You don't have to drink wheat grass juice or even install an anti-McDonald's detection device on your car, as much as both of those might be a good idea. You don't have to become a health nut, spend hours in a gym or sit in the lotus posture chanting "Om."

This 46-page book is an immediate action guide filled with common sense ideas proven in thousands of published medical studies to prevent, reverse and, yes, even cure many diseases. None of us wants to be sick, disabled, in pain or old before our time. More importantly, none of us wants this for our children and grandchildren.

Everything will change when you realize that you have the power and information to begin the world over again, as Thomas Paine said.

The most important asset you have in your life is your good health. Without it, nothing else matters.

Chapter 2
Foods that heal, foods that kill

I am passionate about healthy food. I abhor the toxic food to which most Americans are addicted.

The food industry has enticed us with thousands of easy-to-use processed food products, loaded with The Terrible Three: sugar/simple carbs, bad fats and salt. The Terrible Three have turned us into a nation of overeaters and fast food/processed food junkies. We love greasy burgers, fries and giant gulps of cola, because they taste good and give us a quick high. They're loaded with The Terrible Three and our palates are conditioned to crave these tastes.

Think about this: Every calorie and every gram of carbohydrate, protein and fat that goes into your body has to go somewhere. You burn calories in your everyday activities, but every extra calorie you consume that is not immediately burned is stored as body fat and leads to diabetes and obesity.

Diabetes and obesity are frequent causes of heart disease, kidney failure, blindness, nerve damage, arthritis and strokes. Most of us consume far more calories than can be immediately burned. Studies prove that for optimal weight and maximum disease-free longevity, we should be eating about 1,200 calories a day, but the average American consumes two to three times that much.

The first thing you need to know about food is that you *must* reduce your calorie intake to achieve your ideal weight. There's no way around it!

Visit **www.naturalcuresmd.com** for free calculators to monitor and track your body mass index and determine your ideal weight.

This chapter consists of two simple lists:

The first is a list of healing foods you should eat every day and why. They are the foods that are the foundation of a healthy life. They are the true natural cures Mother Nature provides. They will protect your cells from the diseases of aging by providing large amounts of antioxidants and nutrients. They can even prevent and reverse many diseases, including heart disease and cancer.

Eat organic foods if you can to reduce the load of toxins, antibiotics, growth hormones, pesticides and herbicides added to most commercially grown food. Eat these foods daily, and they will reward you with a vigorous, healthy and happy disease-free long life.

The second is a list of foods that kill. They kill because they replace the life-giving foods that heal and they overload your body with toxic soup of bad fats, chemicals and sugars. Sadly, they are foods that almost all Americans consume nearly every day. It's time for you to renounce them. Save your life and opt for life-giving foods rather than life-destroying foods. If you make the choice to eat from this list, do so extremely sparingly and with the awareness that you are quite literally shortening your life every time you do so. They are just as harmful as smoking, which can take 20 years or more off your life. And just like smoking, these foods that kill cause heart disease, strokes and cancer.

FOODS THAT HEAL

Broccoli and other cruciferous vegetables

Broccoli may be the single biggest health protector you can put on your plate. It's loaded with some of the most powerful nutrients known to science, proven to prevent and cure the diseases of aging.

Just think about those sulphorophanes in broccoli that can cut the risk of various types of cancer in half if you eat four servings a week; indole-3-carbinol will detoxify and usher free estrogens out of your system, which can combat hormonally related cancers.

This is not a political statement, but let me just say for the record that when the first President Bush whined about hating broccoli, he did a great disservice to himself and to his constituents. Broccoli is one of the best things you can give your body. Eat it every day and teach your children to love it!

Try these other cruciferous vegetables with similar benefits: cauliflower, cabbage and Brussels sprouts.

Berries

If broccoli is the king of vegetables, berries hold an equally prominent position in the fruit world. Blueberries are at the top of the antioxidant scale for fresh fruits. Blackberries, strawberries, raspberries and cranberries are loaded with antioxidants that neutralize harmful free radicals that cause damage to your cells. This free radical damage leads to cancer, heart disease, dementia and even arthritis. Studies on blueberries indicate they can also improve memory.

These vibrantly colored fruits are the best possible sources of flavonoids. Flavonoids are powerhouse antioxidants that promote healthy cell growth and prevent cellular mutations that can become cancerous. Research suggests that a diet rich in flavonoids may significantly reduce your risk of many deadly forms of cancer.

The blue-purple color of blueberries, blackberries and raspberries comes from anthocyanadin, a particularly powerful type of flavonoid known to strengthen cells against the deterioration of day-to-day living.

Apples

Apples are packed with two of the most powerful antioxidants known: quercetin and ellagic acid. Apples also contain a plethora of phenolic and flavonoid compounds that are proven disease fighters. Pectin in apples helps sweep toxins from your system. These two disease-fighting superheroes have been shown to reduce LDL "bad" cholesterol by up to 34 percent. Another study showed that people who ate the most apples had a reduced risk of lung cancer. Quercetin and ellagic acid also prevent collagen breakdown, keeping skin firmer and joints stronger. Studies on quercetin indicate those who consume the highest levels have about 50 percent less risk of heart disease and strokes.

There's more: Apples are a key dietary source of boron, a mineral that studies suggest helps women maintain estrogen levels during menopause and may help reduce bone loss.

Apples provide a fat-free, cholesterol-free, sodium-free, low-calorie (80 calories per medium apple) treat that gives you plenty of fiber to help clean your digestive tract. You'll get five grams if you eat the whole fruit, skin and all.

Spinach and other dark green leafy vegetables

These vegetables are packed with a wide variety of nutrients ranging from vitamin A to estrogen-inhibiting indoles and other flavonoids to fiber that signal your liver to turn up the production of enzymes that break down cancer-causing toxins.

Several studies have proven the nutrients in dark green veggies attack several types of cancer cells—especially those in the breast, cervix, prostate and urinary tract—and may reduce the risk of these cancers.

Excellent sources of vitamins C and A, folate and magnesium, dark green leafy vegetables help keep arteries clear, lower blood pressure, strengthen heart muscle and lower levels of homocysteine, a risk factor for heart attacks and stroke.

Want more reasons to fill your plate or salad bowl with spinach? Spinach is a great source of bone-strengthening vitamin K, calcium and magnesium. It also has several anti-inflammatory compounds that protect against arthritis and asthma as well as lutein to protect eyesight and reverse macular degeneration. Studies indicate cooked spinach is actually more beneficial than raw spinach. I recommend lightly sautéing it with organic extra virgin olive oil and organic garlic to help protect against vision loss, heart disease and even cancer!

Other vegetables with similar benefits: kale, Swiss chard and collard greens.

Coldwater wild-caught fish

Salmon, tuna, trout, sardines and mackerel are the best known sources of the omega-3 fatty acids EPA & DHA. These essential fats protect your heart, your cells and your mental function—and help you lose weight. Studies indicate that depression can be alleviated with adequate intake of omega-3 fatty acids. Omega-3s are also powerful anti-inflammatory nutrients and can ameliorate arthritis pain.

A recent Australian study found that a daily serving of salmon, mackerel or sardines helped subjects lose weight by decreasing blood levels of the messenger hormone leptin by an impressive 80 percent, shutting down the body's fat-storing machinery.

Be sure you get wild-caught fish because farm-raised fish fed a high-grain diet lose their high omega-3 content and they may have high levels of mercury and other heavy metal toxins. I personally recommend Wild Planet's minimal mercury tuna and salmon. It has a fraction of the level of mercury and much higher levels of omega-3s compared to typical store-bought brands.

Not a big fan of fish? No problem! You can do just as well without the mercury risk by getting your omega-3 fatty acids from molecularly distilled fish oil supplements.

Olive oil and other healthy oils

Olive oil is loaded with antioxidants and healthy monounsaturated fats. Versatility in cooking and for dressings combined with its great taste make olive oil my number 1 choice for a healthy fat. People who use olive oil regularly, especially in place of other fats, have much lower rates of heart disease, atherosclerosis, diabetes, colon cancer and asthma. Olive oil is one of the main ingredients of the heart-healthy Mediterranean diet, an eating plan proven to be far superior to most other dietary programs. I strongly recommend organic extra virgin olive oil as your first choice for a healthy fat in salad dressing and sautéing. Rice bran oil is another good choice and also contains powerful antioxidants called tocotrienols.

Whole grain bread and pasta

100 percent whole grain (wheat) breads, cereals and pasta products literally scour out clogged arteries, lower cholesterol, help control blood sugars and keep weight in check.

Harvard research showed women who ate the most whole grains reduced their risk of heart disease by a substantial 33 percent.

Add oatmeal to this list for its heart protective benefits. The water soluble fiber in oatmeal acts like chewing gum: It gets very sticky and literally attaches itself to cholesterol molecules, sweeping them out of your body before they can trigger plaque buildup in your arteries. These foods are high in fiber, a powerful ingredient in the fight against heart disease, diabetes and cancer.

Beans and lentils

All beans and lentils are excellent sources of fiber and antioxidants. Daily consumption helps keep blood sugar under control and may be a natural remedy for diabetes. This is especially important considering the 15 million Americans with diabetes and millions more with elevated glucose and insulin that leads to heart attacks, stroke and blindness.

Although they are high in complex carbohydrates, beans and lentils are also high in protein and they're low on the glycemic index scale because the protein and fiber helps balance the carbs. So eat them freely as a food that heals.

Black beans are as rich in antioxidant compounds called anthocyanins as grapes and cranberries, fruits long considered antioxidant superstars. When researchers analyzed different types of beans, they found that the darker the bean's seed coat, the higher its level of antioxidant activity. Ounce for ounce, black beans have the most antioxidant activity, followed by red, brown, yellow, and white beans. Overall, the level of antioxidants found in black beans is approximately 10 times that found in an equivalent amount of oranges and comparable to that found in grapes or cranberries.

Tomatoes (cooked)

Lycopene is a unique and powerful carotenoid that gives tomatoes red color and can lower the risk of certain cancers, including breast and cervical cancer.

In one study, women with the highest lycopene intake had a 45 percent lower risk of breast cancer. Lab research suggests lycopene inhibits growth of breast cancer cells by 88 percent. Lycopene has also been shown to decrease risk of prostate, ovarian, endometrial, lung, colon and pancreatic cancers. Studies also show lycopene is a natural prostate cancer remedy since it reduces the risk dramatically and may even prevent progression after cancer has already occurred.

Eating just two tablespoons of tomato paste daily can lower LDL cholesterol by up to 23 percent and a serving of cooked tomatoes a day can reduce your risk of a heart attack and heart disease by 30 percent.

Lycopene's antioxidant shield against free radicals extends to brain cells, possibly preventing cell damage that eventually leads to memory loss.

Eat your tomatoes cooked because heat breaks down the cell walls and makes the lycopene more available to your body. The longer they are cooked, the better. It also helps if you add olive oil or rice bran oil since lycopene is a fat-soluble nutrient and needs fat for absorption.

Other high lycopene foods: All tomato products, watermelon, pink grapefruit, guava and apricots.

Mushrooms

Symbols of longevity in Asia because of their health-promoting properties, the Chinese have used shiitake mushrooms medicinally for thousands of years. Shiitake mushrooms contain a polysaccharide called lentinan that boosts immune system function, revving up your body's ability to fight off everything from colds and flu to AIDS. Lentinan is also credited with powerful cancer protective properties. It seems to work by seeking out cancerous cells and tumors and killing them.

Several animal studies conducted over the last ten years show eritadenine, an enzyme found in shiitake mushrooms, lowered cholesterol levels regardless of the types of dietary fats the lab animals were given.

Other nutritious mushrooms: reishi, maitake and cordyceps.

Garlic and onions

Regularly eating onions and garlic can reduce the risk of stomach, colon and breast cancers—even if you eat as little as one slice of raw onion a day.

The combination of sulfur and quercetin in onions neutralizes nitrosamines, which are among the most virulent naturally occurring causes of cancer in the human body. Studies published on garlic indicate it can lower cholesterol, reduce artery-clogging plaque in just six months and reverse aging of the aorta. Garlic is also a powerful natural remedy against viruses and bacteria.

Lean meats and poultry

I'll bet you never thought I'd recommend eating meat, and red meat at that, but here it is: Lean grass fed (preferably organic) red meat is the best source of conjugated linoleic acid (CLA, a powerful nutrient that helps control weight and may even be an anti-cancer agent). CLA reduces fat storage and sends fats to the muscles to be burned for energy, thereby increasing the calorie-burning abilities of the lean muscle mass. It specifically targets dangerous belly fat. Typical store-bought steaks are not derived from grass-fed cattle, so be sure to choose free range and organic wherever possible. Also, it is important to select the lean cuts such as sirloin and strips to avoid excess fat. Even with this said, try to limit your red meat intake to no more than once a week. Another option for increasing your CLA consumption is a supplement called Tonalin.

Of course, all animal products are good sources of complete proteins. You can get 67 percent of your body's daily protein needs in just four ounces of chicken (free-range, organic, of course). Chicken is also a good source of selenium, another powerful anti-cancer nutrient.

Red wine

Drinking moderate amounts of red wine can literally save your life and certainly will extend it. Prestigious research institutions like Harvard and M.D. Anderson Cancer Center say resveratrol, the compound in the skins of red grapes, literally taps into the longevity gene.

For more than 70 years, research has proven that near-starvation diets result in longer life. But who wants to do that? A recently identified enzyme called SIR2 works the same magic, without the dire calorie restriction. Resveratrol activates SIR2, increasing the lifespan of virtually every species studied by up to 60 percent—and theoretically there's no reason to believe why it couldn't have some benefit for humans.

Resveratrol is very similar to estrogen in chemical structure. It can bind to estrogen receptors and put an end to annoying symptoms of perimenopause like hot flashes and insomnia.

On a deeper level, resveratrol can neutralize free estrogen molecules that cause all sorts of havoc ranging from heart disease to breast cancer. Lab studies suggest that resveratrol may significantly lower the risk of breast, colon, skin and other forms of cancer. What's more, researchers suggest getting resveratrol in their teens and early 20s can actually "inoculate" women against many future cancers.

Finally, sipping a glass of red wine a day reduces the risk of heart attack by as much as 52 percent by keeping arteries more elastic and working as a powerful heart protective inflammation fighter.

Green tea

This amazing beverage contains EGCG (epigallocatechin gallate), a powerful antioxidant proven in numerous studies to force cancer cells to literally commit suicide, a process called apoptosis. Studies show that EGCG can even kill strains of flu. Finally, green tea's antioxidants keep your cells strong and young.

They can even help increase your metabolism, making it is a good tool for weight loss.

Other teas

Black and white teas come from the same plant as green tea, they're just processed slightly differently. Green tea is the best, but black and white teas are worth including in your new eating plan.

Dark chocolate

Consume only quality, preferably organic, dark chocolate. None of that high-sugar candy with a very low cocoa content. Go for the *real* dark stuff (55–70 percent cocoa) for real heart protection, mood improvement and long life.

Nothing boosts your brain's levels of the feel-good hormones, serotonin and dopamine, like chocolate. Recent research shows it's also packed with heart-protecting and cancer-fighting antioxidants including magnesium, polyphenols, arginine and mood-boosting xantines. It also contains phenylethylamine, an antioxidant that has been shown to lower LDL cholesterol by 8 percent and raise HDL cholesterol by 4 percent.

Nuts

Most nuts, especially almonds and walnuts, are great for your heart. They help lower cholesterol, reduce your risk of stroke, and relax hardening arteries. The high levels of magnesium act as natural heart protective calcium channel blockers. One very large study showed that women who substituted nuts for a serving of high-carb foods daily reduced their risk of heart disease by 30 percent. The high levels of magnesium, potassium, manganese, riboflavin and copper in nuts fuel your body's energy-producing furnaces, leaving you energetic and calm.

Water

This treasured liquid is truly the stuff of life. Drink 64 – 96 ounces per day. Water is the second most important nutrient for life, just after oxygen. More than two-thirds of your body is made up of water, and your brain is nearly 75 percent water.

Municipal water supplies contain chlorine and other possible toxins, so it's best to avoid unfiltered tap water. A sink filter or a whole house filter will render this precious nutrient clear, sparkling and healthy, or you may opt for bottled spring water.

Experts estimate that 75 percent of us don't drink enough water, and one study shows just a 2 percent drop in the water in your body may be a cause of fuzzy thinking and daytime fatigue. Dehydration can also lead to urinary tract infections and constipation.

In fact water and fiber are the two most potent natural cures for constipation!

Note: Eat all of these foods as close to their natural form as possible. If you can go organic, by all means, do so to avoid herbicides, pesticides, antibiotics, growth hormones and other harmful substances. If you can't get fresh fruits or vegetables, go for frozen. Canned goods (with the exception of fish, tomato products, beans and legumes) have had virtually all their nutrients cooked out, so avoid them.

FOODS THAT KILL

OK, here it is: my diatribe. These are foods that are absolutely-positively-no-doubt-guaranteed to cause disease, disable you and even kill you. I call them killer foods for a reason. Don't eat them!

Most of them are loaded with one, two or all of The Terrible Three: saturated and trans fats, sugar/refined flours and sodium. They have little to zero nutritional value and even worse, they are toxic.

They are universally high in calories that lead to diabetes and obesity while being devoid of the life-saving fiber, amino acids, antioxidants, healthy fats, vitamins and minerals that your body requires to stay healthy and disease free.

They clog up your arteries and overload your pancreas so your body stops balancing its sugars properly.

They cause cancer, depression, heart disease and shorten your life. They are killers!

I'm going to be brief here because you already know why these foods are bad. Sadly, our taste buds have been conditioned to believe these things taste good, so we want more.

I recommend you *never* indulge in these killer foods, but if you do, please, for your own sake, make your indulgences very rare.

Sugar

Sugar is right at the top of the list of killer foods. There is literally none worse. More than 70 studies define how sugar kills: by suppressing the immune system, increasing cholesterol, feeding cancer cells, potentially triggering autoimmune diseases, causing obesity and premature aging. I can't urge you strongly enough to stay away from sugar. It has many hidden names including high fructose corn syrup utilized in soda.

The average American eats more than 200 pounds of sugar a year, compared to just four pounds a year a century ago—a 50-fold increase. If that doesn't scare you, nothing will. It is no accident this increased sugar consumption parallels the increased obesity rate!

Part of the problem is that sugar is a hidden ingredient in many foods—but a bigger part of the problem is that our collective sweet tooth is out of control and it's driving us into early graves.

Sodas (including diet)

The average 16-ounce soda has 12 teaspoons of sugar and 180 calories. But let's get real here: Who drinks just a 16-ounce Coke these days? I remember in my boyhood when a Coke was 8 ounces. Now the convenience store sells 64-ounce Big Gulps and the fast food outlets have unlimited free refills. So let's think of the average soft drink lover getting 360 calories and 24 teaspoons of sugar per guzzling session—or more. The average American drinks an appalling 56 gallons of soft drinks a year.

Not only do soft drinks make you fat, they have been linked to osteoporosis, tooth decay and heart disease.

You like diet soft drinks? Forget it. They don't have the sugar or the calories, but they're loaded with chemicals, and recent research links them to an increased risk of obesity, probably because folks are super-sizing and thinking they're making a healthier choice by choosing a diet drink. Studies indicate the artificial sweetener aspartame used in many diet sodas may be a neurotoxin and destroy brain cells. A recent study indicated high consumption of cola drinks, including diet colas, increases your risk of high blood pressure.

Eliminating or at least drastically reducing all types of soft drinks from your diet may be the simplest and most important health choice you can make. Replace them with green tea made with spring water for a natural cure for obesity and other diseases.

Trans fatty acids

No amount of trans fatty acids, not even the tiniest bit, is acceptable in the human diet. Yet they're in most of the snack and fried foods we love most. The process of hydrogenation that makes the fats solid and gives them long shelf-life also destroys all the healthy essential fatty acids and forms many toxins. Many processed foods and most fast foods are sources of these killer fats.

Several studies confirm that trans fatty acids (also known as hydrogenated or partially hydrogenated vegetable oils) raise LDL "bad" cholesterol and drop HDL "good" cholesterol dramatically and they reduce elasticity of arteries. This all adds up to a huge risk of heart disease. Other studies indicate trans fatty acids increase cancer risk.

Some of the main culprits are stick margarine, commercial cookies and baked goods, chips, french fries and other fried snack foods.

French fries

Artery-clogging death sticks—that's what I call them. They're saturated with grease, and usually trans fatty acids. The potatoes themselves are full of simple carbs, and, as if this was not bad enough, when you drown them in grease they become especially lethal. One large order of fast food french fries has an appalling 6 grams of trans fat. If you want potatoes, don't fry them, drown them in butter or drench them with sour cream. A baked potato with salsa or yogurt on top or a helping of oven fries made with a minimal amount of olive oil and spices is fine—once in a while.

Deep fried fish or deep fried anything for that matter

I'm still harping on trans fats and frying with vegetable oils, but I won't apologize. By drowning your healthy fish in grease, you're destroying all the essential fatty acids. Studies prove that fried fish is toxic and harmful, increasing disease rates. Don't do it! If you must fry, use rice bran oil. It's far less harmful than frying with vegetable oils.

Refined grains (white bread, pasta, cookies, cakes, etc.)

Highly refined flour has virtually no nutritional value, no fiber and virtually all vitamins and minerals are destroyed in the refining process. Worse yet, refined flour can cause carbohydrate imbalances and even alter insulin production. It is the same as eating sugar. Pretty much the same is true for white rice, which has had most of its nutrients removed in the polishing process.

White breads and pastas have little taste. Opt for 100 percent whole grain and brown rice for better taste and far better nutrition.

Donuts

These are a triple killer threat, a gourmand's paradise of The Terrible Three. They're made of no-nutrient white flour, drenched in toxic grease and doused with sugar and sodium. The average donut has more than 300 calories, 17 grams of fat and 33 grams of carbs, half of them sugar. If you have ever made a taste comparison between Dunkin' Donuts and Krispy Kremes, the flower of the South, you know that Krispy Kremes are all this nutritional horror doubled: more fat, more sugar and they feel like a rock in your stomach for three days. Yuck!

Donuts are a guaranteed quick, cheap and tasty way to cause heart disease, cancer, obesity, diabetes and early death.

Bacon, sausage, ham, lunch meat

These cured meats contain nitrates and nitrites, toxic chemicals that can develop into cancer-causing nitrosamines in the body. For example, the nitrosamines in bacon have been shown to increase the risk of pancreatic cancer by 67 percent. Other studies have indicated nitrosamines increase cancer risk by over 1,000 percent. Even more shocking, kids who eat hot dogs drastically increase their risk of leukemia. There is some evidence that consuming vitamin C at high dosages simultaneously with these foods may protect you from these toxins.

I'm not done yet—these same processed meats are high in artery-clogging saturated fat and loaded with additives and colorings that may, in themselves, cause cancer and heart disease. And don't forget the blood pressure-raising sodium that is added at many times the healthy levels we need.

That's it. Not that bad, was it?

You'll notice that the list of foods that heal is much longer than the list of foods that kill. And if you expand it, you'll realize that virtually every vegetable, fruit, legume and nut is life giving. Your choices of foods are huge. If you simply avoid the "foods that kill" list and all things made with them, you've made a giant step toward glowing good health, reducing your risk of heart disease, cancer, dementia, arthritis, obesity, depression and diabetes.

Your body has amazing natural healing power if you support it with the food and nutrients it needs to stay healthy.

Chapter 3
Supplements to add years to your life

Most of us, including the health care professionals who advise us, believe food is the best source of nutrients, but the truth is that none of us eat an optimal diet all the time. Worse yet, our soils have become so depleted that plants cannot extract all the vital minerals as they once did.

Numerous studies prove that diet alone cannot give you the blood levels of many essential nutrients you need to prevent disease, much less to cure it.

Coenzyme Q10 (CoQ10) is a great example of this nutritional shortfall. The average American's diet provides only about 1 milligram (mg) of CoQ10 a day, yet to effectively slow Parkinson's disease, you must consume 400–1,200 mg—400 to 1,200 times the amount you're getting in food!

That means that even if you are eating the freshest, best, organically grown produce, you're still not getting all the nutrients at optimal levels you need.

No, this absolutely does not mean you need to take handful after handful of supplements several times a day. This may sound strange coming from a doctor who has devoted a great deal of his professional life to vitamin research and creating the best possible supplements to maintain health and benefit a wide variety of conditions. That's exactly why I have compiled this list of essential and powerful antioxidant nutrients that everyone needs every day for ideal health.

In truth, you need a top-quality multi-vitamin/mineral/ antioxidant and if you have a specific health concern or disease, you may need a few other supplements. Some top-quality multis may even contain almost everything on this list, so you'll need to spend some time checking labels so you don't duplicate. I also recommend capsules whenever possible for quicker and better absorption, plus they are easier to swallow. A few nutrients, such as SAMe and NADH, need to be in tablet form because of stability issues.

If you have a specific disease condition, like heart disease or diabetes, you'll need to consume more supplements compared to someone who is healthy. This list is basic for folks who are generally healthy and want to remain that way.

Your optimal multi-vitamin/mineral/antioxidant formulation

Even the anti-supplement American Medical Association recommends a multi-vitamin for every man, woman and child for exactly the same reasons I've laid out here: We simply aren't getting the nutrition we need from our food. What I consider the best dose is often far beyond the government's recommended levels (RDA/DV), which are woefully low in most cases.

A top-quality basic multi-vitamin should include:
* Betatene (natural carotenoids)   5,000 – 25,000 IU
* Vitamin B1 (thiamine)   50 – 200 mg
* Vitamin B2 (riboflavin)   10 – 20 mg
* Vitamin B3 (niacinamide)   100 – 200 mg
* Vitamin B5 (pantothenic acid)   10 – 200 mg
* Vitamin B6 (pyridoxine)   50 – 100 mg
* Vitamin B12 (methylcobalamin)   500 mcg – 5 mg
* Folic acid   800 mcg – 5 mg
* Biotin   500 mcg – 5 mg
* Vitamin C (Ester-C®)   500 – 2,000 mg
* Vitamin D   700 – 2,000 IU
* Vitamin E (D-alpha succinate)   100 – 2,000 IU
* Coenzyme Q10   10 – 1,200 mg
* Calcium (citrate malate)   500 – 1,300 mg
* Magnesium   250 – 500 mg
* Zinc (L-OptiZinc®)   15 – 30 mg
* Copper   1 – 2 mg
* Manganese   1 – 2 mg
* Boron   1 – 3 mg
* Selenium (selenomethionine)   200 – 400 mcg
* Chromium   200 – 500 mcg
* Lutein (FloraGLO®)   6 – 20 mg
* Bioflavonoids (quercetin is best)   100 mg – 500 mg
* Alpha Lipoic Acid   150 mg – 1,200 mg
* Grape Seed and
  Green Tea Antioxidants   50 mg – 500 mg

I have included ranges that are based on published studies showing benefits in humans through supplementation. Most of these levels cannot be obtained from diet alone. The lower ranges can be obtained from one or two capsules per day, depending on the product, while the higher ranges require you to consume about six to eight capsules per day.

Some of the nutrients mentioned here may be very familiar to you and you may never have heard of others. Please check the label of your multi-vitamin products carefully to see what's included and then add what else is missing to achieve these optimal levels. The typical "once per day rock hard, complete A to Z vitamin tablet" is missing many of these life-saving nutrients and the ones included in these inferior products are generally well below the optimal range and some cannot even be absorbed by the human body. You're likely to be sorely disappointed when you compare your multi-vitamin label on the cheapies to the list on the previous page.

Most multi-vitamins are horribly inadequate to meet your nutritional needs. In fact, the most popular only costs the manufacturer about two cents per tablet to produce! What can you buy that is worth having that costs two cents? The answer is NOTHING! I strongly recommend you spend a small amount of your annual budget and actually get real protection and benefits. The cost should only be around $1 to $2 per day for good health!

B-complex vitamins

The eight unique nutrients in the B-vitamin group include B1 (thiamine), B2 (riboflavin), B3 (niacin or niacinamide), B5 (pantothenic acid), B6 (pyridoxine), biotin, B12 (methylcobalamin in its most active form), and folate or folic acid.

B vitamins are essential to energy production and proper nerve function. Individual B vitamins have additional functions:

^Thiamine is essential to proper heart function, cognitive function and maintenance of muscle mass. Take 50 to 200 mg a day.

*Riboflavin helps maintain skin integrity and has also been used to treat migraines and sickle cell anemia. Take 10 to 20 mg a day.

* Niacin has anti-inflammatory properties, helps prevent diabetes and in large dosages, lowers cholesterol. Take 100 to 200 mg a day.

* B5 plays an important role in energy production and in the manufacturing of certain hormones and it may also help lower cholesterol. Take 10 to 200 mg a day.

* B6, one of the single most important nutrients in the human body, helps promote many enzymatic reactions, and is involved with communication between the nervous system and virtually every other part of your body. B6 is also used to treat asthma, heart disease, peripheral nerve disease, depression, pre-menstrual syndrome and carpal tunnel syndrome. It is also essential to optimal immune function and hormone balance. Take 50 to 100 mg a day.

* Biotin maintains healthy hair and nails and may have some benefits for diabetics. Take 500 mcg to 5 mg a day.

* B12 is a critical element of proper heart function and along with B6 and folic acid, it lowers levels of homocysteine. Elevated levels of homocysteine may be more dangerous than elevated cholesterol and cause heart attacks, stroke and even Alzheimer's and dementia. Take your B12 in the active methylcobalamin form, as a capsule that actually achieves blood levels similar to B12 injections. This form does not need to be dissolved under the tongue. Take 500 mcg to 5 mg a day.

* Folic acid can help lower blood pressure and homocysteine and it helps prevent certain types of birth defects and even cancer. Take 800 mcg to 5 mg a day.

If your multi doesn't contain these B vitamins in these dosages, you can take a B complex formulation, but be sure the formulation is properly balanced as listed in the multivitamin formula above.

Flavonoids and carotenoids

These plant pigments give many fruits and vegetables their bright colors and work as powerful antioxidants that help prevent the cell damage that leads to a wide variety of the chronic diseases of aging. While they are not considered essential nutrients, some flavonoids support health by strengthening capillaries and other connective tissue and some function to reduce inflammation, minimize allergic reactions and combat viruses. Animal studies at the University of Scranton showed that high doses of flavonoids can reduce the risk of atheroscelerosis over 60 percent.

There's more. Flavonoids have been shown to shut down the production of inflammatory agents that cause allergies. One Japanese study showed an over-the-counter flavonoid preparation was more effective than prednisone, the most commonly used anti-asthma prescription drug. And even more: Flavonoids have been shown to give relief from menopausal hot flashes, reduce the risk of cataracts and they're effective against a wide variety of viruses, including flu and the herpes simplex virus that causes cold sores and shingles.

Green tea, grape seed and red wine contain flavonoids with well documented antioxidant properties and are considered among the most important anti-aging nutrients you can find. Their powerful antioxidant action protects against heart disease and numerous types of cancer. Remember, 80 percent of Americans will suffer and die prematurely from heart disease or cancer. Red grapes and grape seed extract and red wine are rich sources of a unique antioxidant called resveratrol. Resveratrol activates an enzyme that has been clinically proven to extend lifespan by up to 60 percent in virtually every species tested. Resveratrol also guards against hormonally related cancers by neutralizing free estrogen molecules. Green tea contains a compound called epigallocatechin (EGCG), shown in laboratory studies to dramatically inhibit and kill cancer cells, kill the flu virus and even increase metabolism and fat-burning abilities.

Look for standardized green tea with at least 45 percent EGCG. I recommend 250 to 500 mg per day. Non-standardized products may contain little, if any, EGCG. I recommend 50 to 500 mg of grape seed. The most effective product with the most studies is ACTIVIN®.

Quercetin is another amazing flavonoid found in onions, garlic, apples, cherries, red wine and green tea. It has been shown to reduce the risk of dying of heart disease by 42 percent. It may keep your heart young in three ways: by lowering your blood pressure, reducing cholesterol and actually dissolving the dangerous clots known to trigger heart attacks and strokes. A recent animal study indicated quercetin can be protective from the deadly effects of the flu virus by restoring antioxidants to the lungs that the flu virus depletes. How can one little flavonoid do so many things? Antioxidants like quercetin keep all cells functioning properly, and they particularly help prevent the inflammation that we know is at the core of cardiovascular disease as well as several other chronic diseases.

I strongly recommend 100 to 500 mg of quercetin per day.

Essential Fatty Acids (EFAs)

These good fats, also known as the omega-3 fatty acids EPA & DHA, are found in fish oil and are of paramount importance to heart and brain health. Many hundreds of studies show the benefits of EFAs, but perhaps the most significant was one published in early 2005, a review of almost 100 double-blinded randomized clinical trials involving 275,000 people. The results were more than impressive: Patients given prescription drugs like the statins (Lipitor®, Zocor®, etc.) lowered their death rate from heart disease by 13 percent, but those who took omega-3 fats lowered theirs by a very impressive 23 percent without the high cost and dangerous side effects. Another recent study presented at the American Heart Association involved 18,645 people and was conducted over 4.5 years. This study indicated adding 1,800 mg of EPA per day to a statin drug will further decrease your risk of adverse heart problems by 19 percent.

EFAs not only lower cholesterol, they appear to help keep heart rhythms regular and stop blood from clotting. Numerous studies in humans indicate omega-3 EFAs may be a cure for some people that have heart arrhythmias. Omega-3s can also be a powerful natural remedy for depression.

Further, omega-3s can be very effective in reducing joint pain. In one study, 50 percent of arthritis sufferers were able to discontinue their prescription medication after taking EFAs, and there are studies that show they may prevent certain types of cancers and prevent cancer from spreading.

If you are not taking an omega-3 fatty acid with high levels of EPA and DHA, I strongly urge you do so immediately.

Take 1,000 to 2,000 mg of EPA & DHA combined daily from a molecularly distilled fish oil supplement.

MINERALS

Most multivitamins will contain some of these essential minerals, but most of them won't contain enough or in the best forms. Frequently, you'll find the additional amounts you need together in one combination supplement. You can get enough potassium and sodium in your diet alone. But most of us get too much sodium and too little potassium. Too little potassium, calcium and magnesium with too much sodium can lead to high blood pressure.

Calcium
Calcium is the most abundant essential mineral in the human body. Of the two to three pounds of calcium contained in the average body, 99 percent is located in the bones and teeth. Calcium is needed to form bones and teeth and is also required for blood clotting, transmission of signals in nerve cells and muscle contraction. The importance of calcium for preventing osteoporosis is probably its best-known role. Calcium can be a powerful natural cure for osteoporosis and may stop progression of bone loss and may even rebuild bone mass in the elderly. Calcium also has a role in the regulation of blood pressure and cholesterol, and it may have some anti-tumor properties. Supplementation with calcium has been shown to reduce the symptoms of PMS. Vitamin D, magnesium and boron are essential to the absorption of calcium, so if you're taking calcium supplements, you'll need to be sure your supplement contains these three.

I recommend at least 500 mg of calcium citrate malate (a highly absorbed form), 250 to 500 mg of magnesium, 700 IU of vitamin D and 1 mg of boron daily.

Magnesium
Aside from helping your body absorb calcium, magnesium

performs several other important functions. It is needed for bone, protein and fatty acid formation, making new cells, activating B vitamins, relaxing muscles, clotting blood and forming adenosine triphosphate (ATP, the energy your body runs on). The secretion and action of insulin also requires magnesium and this vital element plays a role in 300 crucial enzymatic reactions that keep your body running properly.

Since magnesium is critical and required for energy function, it's not surprising that many people with Chronic Fatigue Syndrome (CFS) and migraine headaches have low magnesium levels. I consider magnesium, combined with CoQ10 and B complex vitamins, to be a natural therapy for many people with migraine headaches and chronic fatigue syndrome. People with diabetes often have low magnesium levels and glucose intolerance and may be corrected with magnesium supplementation. Almost two-thirds of patients in intensive care units are found to be magnesium deficient, suggesting that physiological stresses of illness deplete the body's magnesium stores.

I recommend magnesium malate as a natural remedy for people with fibromyalgia at 500 mg per day. Most people should take 250 to 500 mg a day.

Selenium

This trace mineral is essential for optimal immune system function. It activates an antioxidant enzyme called glutathione peroxidase, which may help protect you against cancer. Yeast-derived forms of selenium have stopped the growth of cancer cells in test tubes and in animals. One study published in the *Journal of the American Medical Association* with over 1,300 subjects showed people who took 200 mcg of selenium in the form of selenomethionine a day for 4.5 years had a 50 percent reduction in their overall cancer death rate and a 37 percent reduction in cases of cancer compared with the placebo group. Another study found that men consuming the most dietary selenium developed 65 percent fewer cases of advanced prostate cancer than men with the lowest levels of selenium intake. Also, studies indicate selenium protects people who have hepatitis and viral infections.

Let me warn you: The typical multi-vitamin has the wrong form of selenium at inadequate levels. I recommend only selenomethionine at 200 to 400 mcg per day for the best proven benefits.

Zinc

This essential mineral is a component of more than 300 enzymes needed to repair wounds, maintain fertility in adults and growth in children, synthesize protein, help cells reproduce, preserve vision, boost immunity and protect against free radical damage. L-OptiZinc® is the best form and has up to 20 times the antioxidant power when compared to other forms of zinc. Zinc lozenges have been proven to reduce the duration of colds in adults.

Take 15 to 30 mg of L-OptiZinc daily, but if you're using it to stave off a cold or sore throat, you can take 25 mg lozenges several times a day for a few days.

Coenzyme Q10

Coenzyme Q10 is a strong ally to help protect you and your cells against premature aging, heart disease, cancer and Parkinson's. This super-powerful antioxidant is like a spark plug in a car's engine. Just as a car cannot function without that initial spark, the human body cannot function without CoQ10. In lab studies, CoQ10 prolonged youth and extended life. It can even be a natural cure for gum disease.

The latest research shows CoQ10 can also help restore failing hearts (congestive heart failure) by increasing cardiac output, slow the brain's aging in Parkinson's disease and possibly protect you against Alzheimer's. Recent Thomas Jefferson University research showed that taking 150 mg of CoQ10 daily cut the number of migraines in half for 61 percent of subjects. CoQ10 is the first product ever proven in humans to actually slow Parkinson's progression—in one study by as much as 50 percent.

CoQ10 works by making every cell as healthy and strong as possible from the inside and protects it from outside attacks. Your body's production of CoQ10 begins to slow in your 20s and by your 40s, your levels could be reduced by half. Plus, your stores may be further depleted if you have heart disease, diabetes, cancer or if you take cholesterol-lowering drugs called statins. A Columbia University study found that Lipitor (a statin drug) can cause a sharp and rapid decline in CoQ10 levels which can actually *cause* heart problems, muscle and nerve damage.

Look for the natural "trans" form of CoQ10 made in Japan. I recommend healthy people and certainly those taking statin drugs take 10 to 200 mg daily. Patients with Parkinson's or heart failure need 400 mg to 1,200 mg per day.

Lycopene

This nutrient gives the red color to tomatoes and acts as one of the most powerful antioxidants known. Multiple studies have shown lycopene can lower the risk of certain hormonally related cancers, including breast, cervical and prostate, by 35 percent or more. A study conducted by Harvard researchers examined the relationship between lycopene and the risk of prostate cancer. Men who got 6.5 mg of lycopene or more in their diets decreased their risk of prostate cancer by 21 percent compared with those who ate the least. Another study indicated that men with prostate cancer who took 30 mg of lycopene per day limited progression of the disease. Other studies indicate lycopene reduces the risk of macular degeneration and heart disease. Take 15 to 30 mg daily in the Lyc-O-Mato® form.

Acetyl-L-Carnitine (ALC)

Some say this amino acid helps turn back the hands of time. That's because it is so important to energy production in your body and for a wide range of functions that help keep you feeling vital and young. It is considered essential in helping to transport fatty acids into mitochondria (the power plants of the cells). It is well-known that individuals can become ALC-deficient for a number of reasons. ALC, aside from being an incredible anti-aging nutrient, also has shown benefit for several medical conditions, including cardiovascular disease, angina and congestive heart failure, liver and kidney disease, peripheral neuropathy, obstructive lung disease and multiple sclerosis. Take 500 to 2,000 mg a day.

Alpha Lipoic Acid (ALA)

ALA, as it is commonly known, often goes hand-in-hand with acetyl-L-carnitine in staving off the effects of aging. Both nutrients have thousands of published studies dating back to the 1950s proving their safety and effectiveness. In fact, one study published in a prestigious medical journal showed that aging rats, when given a combination of both acetyl-L-carnitine and alpha lipoic acid, began performing more like younger rats. When these animals were autopsied, they actually found regeneration of parts of the brain, showing ALA and ALC to be among the most powerful anti-aging compounds known.

On its own, ALA is known as the universal antioxidant because it is capable of regenerating several other antioxidants back to their active states, including vitamin C, vitamin E, glutathione and coenzyme Q10, spreading these original antioxidants' considerable benefits to virtually every body system. ALA is a water- and fat- soluble antioxidant, so it protects cells from the inside and the outside.

ALA can help improve glucose usage in people with diabetes. It can help reverse nerve damage in diabetics and prevent the formation of the most damaging free radicals that lead to many of the complications of diabetes. Take 150 to 1,200 mg per day.

Lutein

This antioxidant found in spinach is in the carotenoid family and is the primary nutrient present in the central area of the retina of your eye, called the macula. Lutein filters potentially damaging forms of light to protect the macula from age-related macular degeneration, the leading cause of blindness in older adults.

One study found that adults with the highest amount of lutein in their diets reduced their risk of macular degeneration by 57 percent compared with those people with the lowest intake. Another study showed a similar link between low dietary lutein and increased risk of cataracts.

In fact, in a study at the Chicago V.A. Hospital, patients with macular degeneration who took lutein daily combined with antioxidants, vitamins and minerals in a formula called OcuPower® actually experienced improved vision with the supplements. Visit www.ocupower.com for more details.

Take 6 to 20 mg daily in the patented and clinically proven FloraGLO® form.

DHEA *(Dehydroepiandrosterone)*

This hormone produced by the adrenal glands is converted into other hormones, including estrogen and testosterone, as your body needs them. Supplementation with DHEA-S (a form of DHEA) resulted in increased levels of testosterone in men, suggesting it may help address problems with erectile dysfunction. Some clinical trials suggest DHEA supplementation lowers fat mass without reducing total body weight, but it appears that effect is more pronounced in men than in women.

Another fountain of youth supplement, DHEA may help increase bone density, sexual desire and skin elasticity. Studies also indicate it helps maintain a healthy immune system as you age. If you're a woman, take 5 to 15 mg daily and if you're a man, the dosage should be 25 to 50 mg a day. If you have any current cancer or cancer risks, you should talk to your doctor about DHEA before taking it. Also it is a good idea to have your DHEA blood levels checked by your doctor to optimize the levels.

OBESITY AND WEIGHT LOSS

Natural cures for obesity and weight loss created by Mother Nature are quite abundant and safe without the toxic effects of diet drugs and ephedra.

My favorites are:

        hoodia gordonii: 500 mg to 750 mg per meal

        CLA (Tonalin®): 1,000 mg per meal

gymnema sylvestre: 500 mg daily
chromium: 200 – 500 mcg daily
5-HTP: 100 – 200 mg daily
green tea: 500 mg a day
glucomannan: 4,000 mg a day
l-carnitine: 1,000 mg daily
calcium pyruvate: 3 to 5 grams a day
fiber: 25 to 35 grams a day
omega-3 EPA & DHA: 2,000 mg a day.

There are numerous published studies proving these are safe and effective nutrients for weight loss and fat burning. Better yet, they are synergistic and work even better when you take them together.

For a free comprehensive weight loss plan, recipes and more supplement details visit www.naturalcuresmd.com/diet.

NATURAL CURES FOR DEFECTIVE JOINTS AND ARTHRITIS

Osteoarthritis (OA), the "wear and tear" deterioration of cartilage in joints as we age, limits mobility for more than 50 million Americans.

Fortunately, there are safe, natural alternatives to the prescription NSAID drugs like the COX-2 inhibitors Vioxx® and Celebrex that turned out to increase the risk of heart disease. Also, all NSAIDs, including aspirin and ibuprofen, can cause gastrointestinal tract bleeding, kidney damage and even death. Tylenol is toxic to the liver and people have died from combining it with alcohol. There are no safe drugs for arthritis, even over-the-counter remedies. Even worse, these NSAIDs may actually increase the progression of joint destruction and lead to joint replacement surgery. Fortunately, Mother Nature has given us some safe and effective natural cures.

Glucosamine sulfate

The best-studied of the natural supplements, glucosamine is very effective in treating arthritis pain and even reversing the damage. There have been a number of studies in the medical literature demonstrating that glucosamine slows and even reverses the deterioration of cartilage in joints. Glucosamine apparently works two ways: by stopping the breakdown of cartilage and by stopping the inflammation cycle.

Take 1,500 mg a day and make sure to use the sulfate form for additional benefits.

Chondroitin sulfate

Chondroitin increases joint mobility, slows cartilage loss and it may actually help to rebuild cartilage. Chondroitin sulfate is naturally present in the human body. It actually attracts water to the cartilage, making it more flexible and at the same time stops the production of enzymes that break down cartilage.

Chondroitin is usually taken with glucosamine. A recent analysis of seven clinical trials indicates that supplementing with chondroitin can reduce osteoarthritis pain by 50 percent.

Take 1,200 mg daily.

Methylsulfonylmethane (MSM)

Sulfur molecules like those found in MSM are essential to the formation of collagen, the joint cushioning molecule. One UCLA study showed subjects with osteoarthritis who took MSM for six weeks reported an 80 percent decrease in pain. Indian research shows that patients with OA who took 500 mg of glucosamine and 500 mg of MSM three times a day for 12 weeks had 63 percent less pain than those who took glucosamine alone and 79 percent less than those who got a placebo, so it is often combined with glucosamine. MSM's benefits seem to be largely through pain relief because of its anti-inflammatory action. MSM also reduces the formation of scar tissue, improves blood flow to the affected joint and may slow the degeneration of cartilage.

I recommend 1,000 to 2,000 mg daily of the OptiMSM® form for the highest quality and purity.

Turmeric

Most of us know turmeric as a culinary herb and the ingredient that gives curry powder its golden color, but this member of the ginger family with potent medicinal properties effectively treats mild osteoarthritis pain and inflammation.

Turmeric's active ingredient, curcumin, is a natural COX-2 inhibitor without unduly suppressing COX-1. Translation: It relieves pain and inflammation without increasing the risk of heart attack and stroke like Celebrex and Vioxx.

Doctors and researchers are unsure exactly how turmeric works, although it appears to inhibit the production of inflammatory chemicals called prostaglandins and leukotrienes. At least two studies, one from the prestigious M.D. Anderson Cancer Center at the University of Texas, showed that turmeric reduced inflammation as powerfully as the prescription drug phenylbutazone (Butazolidine). One Thai study suggests the active ingredients in turmeric suppress the overproduction of inflammation-causing nitric oxide. Numerous studies also indicate turmeric reduces the risk of cancer and even kills cancer cells. Finally, turmeric is a very powerful antioxidant and protects cells from damaging free radicals as we age.

Look for a product standardized 90 to 95 percent curcumins. I recommend 900 to 1,800 mg per day.

Chapter 4
Your quick and easy
30-minute exercise plan

Exercise is one of the most powerful single ways to a long, healthy and happy life.

No, you don't have to spend hours in a gym. In fact, 30 to 45 minutes every other day is really all you need.

EXCUSES

I know you've got a dozen reasons why you can't exercise and right up at the top of the list is, "I don't have time." Am I right?

Other reasons not to exercise: no energy, no place to do it, no money for a fancy gym. Sound familiar?

I'll answer these excuses one at a time:

No time
You can always make time. Get up half an hour earlier. Divide your exercise time (that counts!) and walk for 15 minutes at lunch time, maybe do some strength training while you watch the evening news. Put a mini-trampoline or an exercise ball in your office and bounce while you're on the phone. Run up and down the stairs for five minutes a couple of times a day. Get off the bus one stop early. You can figure this out. You'll actually find you have more time in your day because the exercise is giving you more energy and mental clarity.

No energy
This is one you'll just have to tough your way through. There are probably several reasons you don't have the energy, and primary among them may be your diet and supplement plan. There's a Catch-22 here: If you don't exercise, you don't have energy to exercise. Sensible exercise builds energy, so grit your teeth and get out there and do it. At the beginning, it may be difficult, but make a solemn pledge to yourself you'll do it regularly without fail for at least a month. You'll be surprised how fast you become addicted to the endorphin high that comes with exercise. Another thought about the "no energy" excuse: You may be depressed. However, exercise is probably the best antidote to depression you can find. Studies have actually shown that exercise can be more effective in lifting depression than prescription anti-depressants.

No place to do it

Face it, this is a lame excuse. If you've got a space three feet square, there are scores of exercise videos you can do, covering virtually every aspect of fitness. If you live in a city, hit the sidewalks. If you live in the country, hit the trails. You don't have to have a room devoted to expensive exercise equipment to get with the program.

No money for a fancy gym

You don't need a fancy gym, spandex workout clothes and designer shoes. The most important piece of equipment is a good pair of shoes. Ask around and find a sporting goods store known for savvy salespeople who can fit you perfectly. You may pay $100 for a really good pair of walking shoes, but they'll last a year. That's less than $2 a week. You can afford it! You can buy an exercise ball and exercise bands for less than $20 at any discount store, and exercise DVDs cost about the same. You can even rent a few and decide which you like best. Check with local high schools or colleges for community-based fitness programs. They're usually $10 a week or less. Hey, that's just a couple of Starbuck's lattes that you didn't need anyway.

THE YESES

OK. Now I've addressed all the "NOs" and you're ready to commit to an exercise program. Right?

But what do you do?

Walk

Right off the bat, I recommend walking. Almost anybody can do it, and you don't need any training or fancy equipment except the good shoes I mentioned in the last section.

Harvard research shows that vigorous walking for half an hour a day can reduce the risk of heart disease by as much as 53 percent.

If you have a disability that prevents you from walking, get creative and find something you can do. Try swimming or use a recumbent bike or an elliptical trainer.

Love it

Is walking enough? It may be if you really enjoy it. That's the catch. Exercise only works if you do it and if you don't love it, you won't do it. For some people going to a gym and comparing lats, pecs, abs and quads is a real inspiration. For others, a solitary early morning walk or a bike ride on a lonely trail is exactly what they need to recharge stress-drained batteries. Find something you love to do. The rest will follow.

Get some guidance

No matter what form of exercise you choose, look for some expert advice. A personal trainer can be invaluable—and just paying for two or three sessions will quickly get you on the right track. If you decide you love mountain biking or inline skating, join a club or look for folks who really know what they're doing. They'll advise you and help prevent injuries and accidents.

Go gently

Yoga, tai chi and chi gong are excellent for flexibility, balance and even conditioning. The amount of exercise you'll get with these gentle Eastern disciplines may surprise you. They're not as easy as they look. Don't shortchange yoga, tai chi and chi gong. They're also excellent methods of stress reduction.

That's it. No long lectures, nothing complicated. Just get out there and move.

Chapter 5
Managing your stress

Unless you live in a cave in the Himalayas, it is impossible to exist in today's world without stress. It's a simple fact of modern existence.

It's not the stress itself, but how you handle it that determines whether you can release and start each day anew. If you can't erase your stress load, you carry it from day to day until you have a toxic accumulation that can override your body's natural abilities to bounce back, keeping stress hormone levels high and suppressing your immune system.

In a nutshell, when you experience stress, whether it's the frustration of being stuck in traffic, an intractable boss, recalcitrant children or an uncooperative spouse, your body responds as our ancestors' did when they encountered a physical threat from an enemy tribe or a wild animal. Stress hormones like adrenaline and cortisol are released, and breath and heart rates increase, sending extra blood sugar to the muscles in preparation to fight or flee from the threat of physical danger.

Today's stress responses rarely are caused by a physical threat, so unlike our ancestors who could kick back and relax once the threat had passed, we keep on being wound up for days, weeks, and even months at a time. In the wild, animals that have been stressed often go through a series of movements to disperse the energy and complete the stress cycle. Modern-day humans seem to have forgotten how to do this, so stress—what some call toxic stress—stays inside us and exacts a very high price.

Toxic stress means you have diminished your body's ability to produce the stress hormones cortisol and DHEA when you need them, so you are less able to respond in an appropriate way to stressors and to end the stress cycle.

The cost of toxic stress is huge. In the short term, it suppresses the immune system, slows metabolism and can cause headaches, fatigue, insomnia, dizziness, heartburn and more. In the long term, it accelerates the aging process, contributes to weight gain, increases the risk of heart disease, cancer and digestive problems and contributes to depression and more stress-inducing emotions that escalate the stress cycle.

OK, it goes without saying that none of us wants this stress and yet none of us can escape the stressors of 21st century life. What do we do?

You can manage your stress. Here are few simple secrets:

Sleep

The vast majority of us get seven hours of sleep a night—or less—and 43 percent have insomnia at least once a week. While science can't tell you why we sleep, a host of physical problems result from lack of sleep, including increased risk of diabetes, heart disease and obesity. Getting eight hours of sleep is essential to long-term health and stress reduction. Make a commitment to do just that. It is also critical that you awaken at the same time every day. For each hour you change your waking time, you ruin your sleep patterns for one day. In order to unwind before going to sleep, I like to read in bed with a soft light (preferably a book reading light). Choose a book that is soothing to the soul and certainly not an action novel. As your eyes become heavy, put down the book and turn off the light without getting out of bed.

Breathe

Start by beginning your day with a few deep breathing exercises. If you've ever taken a yoga class, you'll know how to do belly breathing. If not, a yoga class (or tai chi or chi gong) is a perfect antidote to stress and great exercise, too. Any time you become aware you're stressed, stop and take half a dozen deep slow breaths through your nose.

Take inventory of what's important and what's not

If you find yourself losing sleep over what your boss said today or the perceived slight a friend made yesterday or the guy who cut you off in traffic last week—don't! Hanging on to these stressors builds your toxic stress load. I like to use a little "test" to determine if it's worth hanging on to these things. I ask myself, "Am I going to remember this in ten years?" For the vast majority of theses stressors, the answer is, "No." If that's the case, drop it. Why carry that load and damage your health? Going just a little bit further, the power of forgiveness is immense and the consequence of carrying grudges is huge. Try to find your way to forgiveness no matter how justified your anger and hurt. In the end, you're only hurting yourself if you carry these feelings.

Active stress management

There are a number of means of actively managing stress, but two are the most effective, in my mind: keeping a "to do" list and making time for yourself. These two go hand-in-hand. If you have to do it, schedule time for a bubble bath, for daily meditation or a walk after dinner. Make yourself a priority in your daily planning and you'll find your stress load will be considerably lightened.

Spirituality

Finally, spirituality in any form is a very important form of stress relief. There have been dozens of studies that show meditation and prayer are potent de-stressors.

Chapter 6
Your immediate action plan

Here's the plan in a nutshell. You can take a week, a month or a year for each step. Once you've completed a step, move on to the next. By the time you finish Step 4, you'll be a whole new healthy person!

STEP 1: *Multis, nix the fast food, processed food, and take a walk.*

Do you eat fast food or processed food several times a week? I'm not telling you to become a vegan overnight. I'm simply asking you, if you cannot eliminate your toxic food intake completely, reduce it—just a little—by one or two meals a week.

And if you have Big Mac attacks on a regular basis, try going for a regular burger (save 280 calories and 70 percent of the fat) or even a Quarter Pounder (save 110 calories and 20 percent of the fat) instead. If you super size, don't. Try splitting an order of fries with a companion and save 275 calories and grams of killer trans fat. Skip the soft drink entirely and go for an unsweetened iced tea high in antioxidants or even water, and save 310 calories.

Just by switching this one meal, you've knocked off 700 calories. Do this five times a week, and you have neutralized one pound of weight gain (3,500 calories). Think of it the other way: One pound of weight loss per week reduces your weight by 52 pounds in a year! If you're still hungry after your meal, eat an apple or a handful of strawberries. Both are fiber rich, low calorie and full of life saving antioxidants. Nuts are also a good snack option since they contain a good balance of protein, fiber, good fats, potassium and magnesium.

If you find you can't resist the fast food restaurants, try a chicken Caesar salad with low-fat dressing—a big (and reasonably healthy) meal for just 340 calories and 14 grams of fat. Another inexpensive and easy option are Stouffer's Lean Cuisine frozen meals. They have a healthy balance of carbs, protein and fat with a small amount of calories; most of them actually taste good! I also love the Genisoy® nutrition bars with their healthy balance of protein, carbs, fat and nutrients. I often have them for my lunch between patient consults if I only have five minutes to eat.

Food action

Cut back fast food and processed food consumption by at least one meal this week. Eliminate these toxic foods entirely, if possible. The most toxic of all are fried foods, so take the pledge to cut back on all fried foods with this step.

Supplement action

Choose a good multi-vitamin and start taking it every day, without fail. I personally recommend the Nutraceutical Sciences Institute's [NSI®] Synergy multi-vitamin line. I have been using and recommending these products for more than 10 years with excellent results. Further, NSI also has hundreds of the best-quality standardized herbs, amino acids and other beneficial nutrients. I am the president and director of the Scientific Advisory Board that carefully formulates the NSI Synergy products according to the latest medical studies. NSI products are available at wholesale prices at **www.vitacost.com/nsi** or you may call for a free catalog **800-793-2601**. You'll find more information on choosing the right supplements in Chapter 3.

Exercise action

The exercise component of this week's plan is just as important as the food changes you are starting to make, but it's easy to do: Take three, brisk 20-minute walks per week. Get a decent pair of walking shoes. Take along a friend, a family member, your dog or all three. Just do it. You'll notice the difference fast.

STEP 2: Conscious eating, full supplementation and more oxygen.

Not a fast food junkie? Congratulations! Are you a snacker? You know how easy it is to sit in front of the TV and chow down an entire bag of Fritos or a quart of ice cream without even thinking about it.

Food action

When you eat, do nothing else but eat. Don't watch TV. Don't read. Don't check your e-mail. Sit at the table. You can carry on a pleasant conversation with your family or friends, but even then, take some quiet time first to appreciate your food, give thanks if that is part of your spiritual tradition, and savor what's in front of you. Instead of snacking on high-carb and high-toxic fat snacks like Fritos®, Ho-Hos®, Ding Dongs® or ice cream, try nuts, celery, broccoli and other healthy items. Studies indicate a serving of nuts will satisfy your hunger much longer than a similar amount of calories from a high-carb chip snack.

Supplement action

Compare your multi-vitamin to the list in Chapter 3, and buy the additional supplements you need for a perfect balance. Start taking them immediately.

Exercise action

Get up off the couch and do something physical during the television commercials whenever you're watching. Calisthenics, bouncing on an exercise ball, using a mini-trampoline or a treadmill, it doesn't matter—just move. Not a TV watcher? Whatever you do during your evening hours, take five minutes every half hour to stretch, jog in place and get your blood circulating. It's a good idea to do this during your work day, too. You can get in a lot of exercise in these little bursts.

STEP 3: *Watch serving sizes, keep taking supplements and check out your bootie.*

Are you a meat and potatoes type?

Food action

If your plate is usually piled with mounds of mashed potatoes, gravy and large chunks of meat, try shrinking your portions by 20 percent and eating a larger salad or adding another low starch veggie to your plate. The best are cabbage, broccoli, cauliflower and spinach. They are full of antioxidants and have low-sugar content. Most of us eat portions that are far larger than we need, and we choose too many high-starch items like bread, corn, pasta and potatoes. Make low-starch vegetables the major food on your plate while still enjoying your favorite foods.

Don't eat after 8 p.m. If your sweet tooth gets the better of you as the evening progresses, try controlling it with an apple.

As your body starts to get back into balance and you become more conscious of what you are putting into it, you'll find your cravings for sugar, salt and fatty foods will diminish and even disappear. Instead, your mouth will water when you think of big, juicy apples or succulent slices of tomato.

Supplement action

Check the list of additional supplements in Chapter 3, buy them and begin taking them.

Exercise action

This is simple. Of course you're continuing your walks and your exercise during commercials. Now take a good look at yourself from all angles in a full length mirror. Naked. Yikes! Do you like what you see? Most likely not. This is not about guilt! This is about action. Let your fingers do the walking—they could use a little exercise, too. Find the name of a personal trainer this week, make a call and make an appointment for next week. That's it!

STEP 4: Go organic and get a little professional advice.

Food action

If you haven't already done so, start buying organic foods as much as possible. I know, they're more expensive, but they are definitely worth it. If you can only add a few organic items to your shopping list, at the very least try to buy organic lettuces and greens, berries and chicken. These are the products with the most toxic ingredients added.

Supplement action

None needed if you're regularly taking all your supplements. You're probably feeling great!

Exercise action

You've got that appointment with the personal trainer this week. Keep up your regular exercise routine—it's a habit by now isn't it? You may have even decided you miss your walks on the "off" days, so you've added in a couple more days or longer walks on weekends. Good for you!

You're already feeling better about yourself, I'm sure, because you've made dozens of healthy choices in the past three weeks.

Now keep that appointment with the personal trainer. Get some professional advice about what you need to do to get into better physical shape and how to do the exercises correctly.

This may be a bit of a stretch financially, but go for it. Think of all the money you're saving on fast food meals! Even if you just do two or three sessions with your personal trainer, you'll be able to devise a routine that's right for you and keep it up on your own. Refer back to the information about exercise in Chapter 4.

🌾 Conclusion

I hope this little book will become your constant companion. Read it again and again, but most importantly, take action! Carry it with you. Loan it to friends and family! Let it become dog-eared with use. That's what it is meant for.

I know you want better health and longevity for you and your family without the high costs and risks of drugs and surgery. I am proud to have the opportunity to help you achieve your goals!

It's as simple as that. There is nothing else you need to do if you follow the guidance I've offered you here. "These are the times that try men's souls" is one of Thomas Paine's most famous quotes and rings true today in so many ways!

I wish you health, happiness and long life.

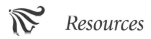 Resources

Due to the fact science and medicine are constantly changing, I've chosen to place references, recommended products and new information on my Web site: www.naturalcuresmd.com. Please visit often!

For more information about Thomas Paine, I recommend the following Web sites:

http://www.ushistory.org/paine/

http://www.thomaspaine.org/

Biography

Dr. Allen S. Josephs is a graduate of Jefferson Medical College in Philadelphia, PA. He completed a three-year residency program in internal medicine at Temple University Hospital in Philadelphia. He then did a second three-year residency in neurology, including serving as chief resident at Mount Sinai Hospital in New York, NY. Since 1984, he has been in private practice in Livingston, NJ. He is also the president and scientific advisory board member of Vitacost.com and has lectured throughout the country to both lay audiences and physicians about the importance of proper nutrition. He was previously appointed by Governor Christine Todd Whitman of NJ to serve as her representative on a medical committee. He is currently the section chief of neurology of St. Barnabas Hospital in Livingston, NJ and co-director of the St. Barnabas Hospital Stroke Center. He is board certified in both internal medicine and neurology.

Acknowledgements

The concept of this book was the brainstorm of Wayne Gorsek, CEO of Vitacost.com. I have known Wayne for about 13 years and he was instrumental in introducing me to the whole realm of nutrition. Since I have known him, he has been my mentor in the matters of nutritional supplementation and a good friend. It is people like him—individuals with great passion and knowledge—who may help to win over the hearts and minds of people in this country to change their way of thinking about their health.

I would also like to thank Ms. Kathleen Barnes for spending many hours in the editing of this book. The hardest part was keeping it to the 46 pages that we had planned. I was fortunate to have Kathleen working on this project, who is extremely well-versed in the field of nutrition. I look forward to working on future endeavors with her.

And of course, I must acknowledge my wife, Marlene, to whom I have been happily married for over 31 years. She has always been supportive in my ventures. We have had a wonderful life together, with hopefully many more years to come.

Finally, I would like to acknowledge the literally tens of thousands of researchers throughout the world who are trying and have been increasingly successful in bringing nutrition to the forefront of scientific investigation for the benefit of all of us.